TOPS CLUB, INC. PRESENTS

THE CHOICE IS YOURS

A practical guide to take off and keep off pounds sensibly

Written By
Ahmed Kissebah, M.D., Ph.D.

with

Howard Rankin, Ph.D.

and

Ann Ruelle, R.D.

Amy Goldwater, B.S.

Illustrations by Jo Anna Poehlman
Line editing by Leah Carson

TOPS Club, Inc., Milwaukee, Wisconsin 53207

Published 1998
Printed in the United States of America

05 04 03 02 01 00 99 98   5 4 3

Publisher's Note:
This publication is designed to provide accurate and authoritative information in regard to the subject matter covered, but with the understanding that TOPS Club, Inc. does not endorse or recommend one brand over another and with the understanding that TOPS Club, Inc. is not engaged in rendering medical or other professional advice. The services of a competent physician or professional person should be sought for medical advice or other assistance. The appearance of any trade name in this publication is not an endorsement or recommendation of that product.

Very rarely do different sources agree completely on the calorie content of specific foods, whether they are natural or processed. Therefore, TOPS Club, Inc. cannot guarantee the accuracy or completeness of the information provided herein. The precise number of calories can only be determined by chemical food analysis, and even this will vary from one batch of a certain food to another. However, in most cases, the variances are not all that striking and are not going to make the difference in successful meal planning and weight loss.

TOPS and KOPS are service marks of TOPS Club, Inc.

ABOUT THE AUTHORS

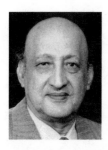

Ahmed H. Kissebah, M.D., Ph.D., F.A.C.P., scientific advisor to TOPS Club, Inc., is internationally recognized as a leader in the study of obesity and related conditions. Dr. Kissebah is a professor of medicine and of pharmacology/toxicology; chief of the Division of Endocrinology, Metabolism, and Clinical Nutrition; and Program Director of the General Clinical Research Center at the Medical College of Wisconsin in Milwaukee, WI. Dr. Kissebah has published many influential scientific papers on his discoveries and is a leader of long standing in many scientific and medical organizations. Dr. Kissebah received his medical degrees at Cairo University in his native Egypt. He earned his Ph.D. at the University of London Royal Postgraduate School in London, England. He also holds an adjunct professorship at Rockefeller University in New York.

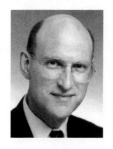

Howard J. Rankin, Ph.D., is a licensed clinical psychologist. An expert on compulsive behaviors, Dr. Rankin has an international reputation in the areas of wellness, eating disorders, and lifestyle change. He has published many scientific journals and has edited several prestigious journals. He has held academic positions at the University of London, where he obtained his masters and doctoral degrees in clinical psychology, and at the University of South Carolina, where he is adjunct professor in the School of Public Health.

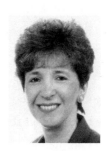

Ann Ruelle, R.D., C.D.E., a registered dietitian and educator, is Director of Nutrition and Diabetic Services for a multi-center medical group in Milwaukee, WI. She is a certified diabetes educator who has served in a number of professional capacities both locally and nationally. Ms. Ruelle has developed nutrition and diabetic programs for radio and television, where she appears regularly. She received her B.S. degree from Mount Mary College in Milwaukee and is a certified lifestyle counselor in the areas of weight and stress management.

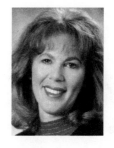

Amy Goldwater, B.S., is a physical fitness expert and educator who leads several programs on fitness and wellness in educational and hospital settings. She received her degree from the University of Michigan, Ann Arbor, and is certified as a fitness specialist through the American Red Cross. Ms. Goldwater is a fitness instructor at a Milwaukee technical college, where she provides training and certification classes for faculty and staff. She is also well recognized for her community outreach programs on wellness and physical activity.

TABLE OF CONTENTS

LISTS OF TABLES AND FIGURES

LIST OF TABLES

LIST OF FIGURES

INTRODUCTION

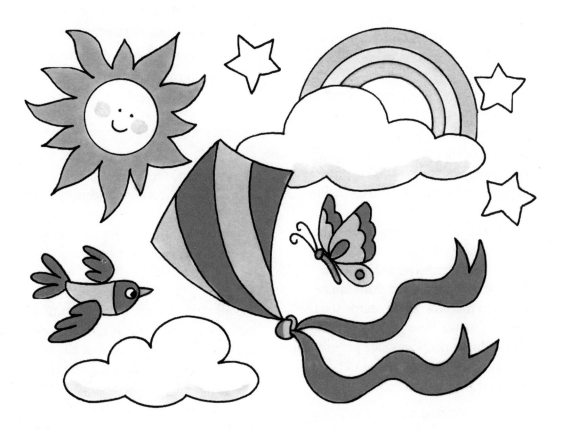

Welcome to the new

TOPS guidebook! This book, written specifically for TOPS members, contains everything you need to lose weight and keep it off. Not only will you find the latest information about nutrition, exercise, medicine, and lifestyle change but also hundreds of great practical tips, fabulous new recipes, and easy-to-do exercises.

In addition to the main guide, we have also included our innovative 28-day program of daily activities that will take you step by step down the path to permanent weight loss. The program is a terrific way to get started and to stay focused on achieving your weight-loss goals. Throughout the guide and the 28-day program, the focus is not just on losing weight but on maintaining your losses, too.

At TOPS, we realize that losing weight and maintaining a healthy lifestyle are not easy tasks. Daily habits cannot be changed overnight or in a week. Change requires continuous effort to make sensible food choices, find the time to exercise, and stay motivated long enough to learn better lifestyle choices. We also recognize that managing your weight concerns more than food; it requires taking control of your life. As a TOPS member, you already have available the most significant resource in your effort to take control of both your weight and your life: the love, support, and experience of your fellow members. Nothing is more powerful than the effect a group of caring individuals can give each other. They give *T*eamwork, *O*penness, *P*erspective, and *S*upport. Information, advice, and skills can be added to this bedrock of interpersonal care to provide a comprehensive program that really works. This guide provides the facts, tips, and advice needed to make weight management a reality.

An ounce of support is worth a pound of information.

Information is important but often is not enough to produce the long-lasting changes in behavior that are necessary for your success. That is why this guide not only includes information but focuses on specific tips, advice, and exercises designed to ensure that you put all this knowledge to good use. This book will enable you to make healthy choices and control your weight.

TOPS FACT:
In the last 14 years, North Americans have become much more informed about nutrition and fitness, yet the number of North Americans considered obese has increased by 33%.

As you will see when you get to the section on motivation, every TOPS member has her or his own reasons for losing weight. It does not matter whether your reasons relate to health, appearance, or self-esteem. Any reason is highly personal, and all reasons are perfectly valid.

It is also true that we are all responsible for our own behavior. Sure, other people can make life difficult for you, but in the final analysis you make your own choices. Every choice you make has a payoff and a price. If you have the facts, you can make an *informed* choice.

This guidebook, therefore, provides facts so that you can make informed choices, and it gives you advice and skills so you can implement those choices.

Each section of the book will give you relevant information and practical advice on how to turn these facts into effective weight-control action. Some sections of the book also provide simple exercises to help you develop specific skills.

There may be a temptation to read only those sections of the book that interest you the most. Please make every effort to read the whole book, for two reasons:
• The book is comprehensive, and many of its sections interconnect.
• The book is written in an entertaining way with many important tips.

While this book is written as a practical guide, it is not designed to make you a health expert.

We also encourage you to take your time going through this guide. There is no need to rush through it. When you rush, you often miss the most important points.

The book is divided into six sections.

The first chapter, *The Medical Perspective,* offers important facts about obesity as well as ways of assessing health risk. It also gives practical tips on the role of your physician and ways of preventing backsliding and yo-yoing.

The *Nutrition and Food Choices* chapter covers valuable information about foods, food labels, and grocery shopping. It contains a comprehensive section on vitamins and minerals and in-depth coverage of both the exchange system and the food guide pyramid. TOPS recommends the exchange system; we have also included the food guide pyramid as a useful visual guide to portion size and good nutrition.

The *Exercise and Physical Fitness* chapter describes how to safely and effectively develop a fitness program that benefits overall health as well as weight. It includes practical tips on how to structure an exercise program, keep it going, and make it enjoyable.

The *Lifestyle Choices and Healthy Behavior* chapter covers such topics as motivation, self-management, craving, bingeing, and managing stress. A weight-management program does not occur in a vacuum, and in this chapter you will find the tools you need to graft your program into your life so that it can really work.

Obesity creates health problems, and in the *Strategies for Special Needs* chapter you will find information and practical advice about common obesity-related illnesses as well as tips for overweight individuals with other special needs.

A *28-day guide* is included to help you start a comprehensive program. It offers a new set of great menus for those trying to maintain weight as well as those trying to lose it.

We hope you not only enjoy this book but find within its pages material that will help you in your efforts to take control. *The choice is yours!*

THE MEDICAL PERSPECTIVE

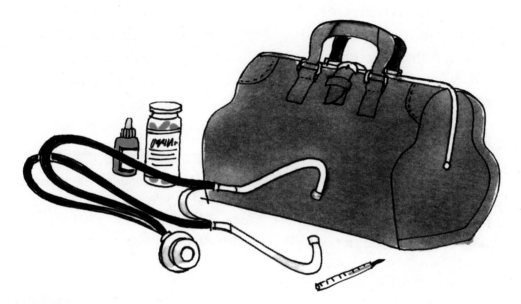

Obesity is both a behavioral and a medical condition. It is important to know about obesity's medical aspects so that you can understand its effects on your health, monitor your progress, make informed lifestyle choices, and keep weight off.

In this section you will learn about the medical aspects of obesity. Specifically, you will learn:

- What obesity is
- How to measure obesity
- Associated health risks
- What causes obesity
- Components of a weight-control program
- The role of your physician
- Available drug and surgical treatments
- What leads to plateaus and yo-yoing

What is obesity?

Fat is a normal part of body composition. Healthy limits for fat are between 15 and 22 percent of body weight for a man and between 18 and 32 percent for a woman. But when the fat levels in your body exceed those limits, you have an excess of fat—and you also have a problem.

IT'S OFFICIAL!
You are officially defined as obese if:
- You are a man and your body fat is greater than 22 percent of your total weight.
- You are a woman and your body fat is greater than 32 percent of your total weight.

Obesity is an Equal Opportunity Employer that affects people from all walks of life. Studies conducted in the U.S., for example, have found 26 million obese men and 32 million obese women. Forty-nine percent of African-American women are obese, as are 22 percent of adolescents. Altogether, about 33 percent of the total U.S. population is obese, and that figure is rising sharply.

Also, based on studies conducted in the U.S., obesity has *increased* by 33 percent in the past decade. In 1984, 25 percent of the population was obese; by the mid-1990s, that figure had jumped to 33 percent. Some people speculate that the increase in obesity is a result of faster paced lives dominated more and more by technology. This leads to lifestyles full of fast food and very little activity. Whatever the reason, the level of obesity has reached epidemic proportions; obesity carries with it some real health dangers.

The dangers of obesity

Obesity is a chronic condition associated with increased disease and mortality risk as well as social and psychological difficulties.

Obesity is associated with four of the major killers in North America. Can you name them? Answers below— and no peeking, please!

Obesity is also associated with impaired qualify of life: decreased mobility, prejudice and discrimination, and damaged relationships, to name but a few factors.

The good news is that even a small weight loss, consistently maintained, can reduce these and other health risks.

DID YOU KNOW?
The health costs of obesity in the U.S. are estimated to be nearly $70 billion annually.

Answers: Obesity is associated with diabetes, high blood pressure, heart disease, and cancer.

Calculating Your BMI

109 980 (handwritten)

You need three things to calculate your BMI:

1. Your weight in pounds   *163* (handwritten)
2. Your height in inches   *65* (handwritten)
3. Your calculator (it doesn't matter how tall or heavy your calculator is)

The Body Mass Index formula is:
weight (pounds) x 705 divided by *height (inches) x height (inches)*

Example:
A woman is 5 feet 5 inches tall and weighs 180 pounds,

Her weight x 705=
180 x 705 = 126,900

height x height =
65 x 65 = 4,225
126,900 divided by 4,225 = 30.04

Her BMI is 30.

If you are using metrics you can calculate your BMI as follows:
weight (kilograms) divided by
height (meters) x height (meters)

27.20   26.3   26.03 (handwritten)

How to determine whether you are obese

If you are uncertain about whether you are officially obese or want to know how obese you are, a simple formula can help you: the Body Mass Index, or BMI. It is a good representative measure of total body fat.

If your calculator is out of batteries or you simply don't want to go through the above exercise, you can find your BMI by consulting the table on the following page.

Once you have calculated a BMI, use the scale below to determine the obesity level that the BMI signifies.

Any BMI greater than 30 is associated with increased health risks.

The woman in our example is just on the edge of the severely obese category. She has just crossed into the BMI territory associated with increased health risks.

Health Risks Associated with BMI Ranges

BMI	Health Risk
27-29.9	moderate
30-34.9	high
35-39.9	very high
40+	extremely high

The BMI Obesity Scale

Category	BMI
Overweight	26-26.9
Obese	27-29.9
Severely obese	30-39.9
Extremely obese	40 or greater

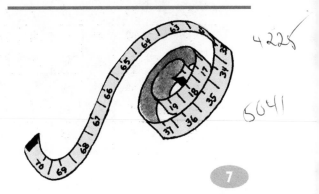

4 225   6641 (handwritten)

Height (feet & inches)

How To Determine BMI

Weight (pounds)	5'0"	5'1"	5'2"	5'3"	5'4"	5'5"	5'6"	5'7"	5'8"	5'9"	5'10"	5'11"	6'0"	6'1"	6'2"
100	20	19	18	18	17	17	16	16	15	15	14	14	14	13	13
105	21	20	19	19	18	17	17	16	16	16	15	15	14	14	13
110	21	21	20	19	19	18	18	17	17	16	16	15	15	15	14
115	22	22	21	20	20	19	19	18	17	17	17	16	16	15	15
120	23	23	22	21	21	20	19	19	18	18	17	17	16	16	15
125	24	24	23	22	21	21	20	20	19	18	18	17	17	16	16
130	25	25	24	23	22	22	21	20	20	19	19	18	18	17	17
135	26	26	25	24	23	22	22	21	21	20	19	19	18	18	17
140	27	26	26	25	24	23	23	22	21	21	20	20	19	18	18
145	28	27	27	26	25	24	23	23	22	21	21	20	20	19	19
150	29	28	27	27	26	25	24	23	23	22	22	21	20	20	19
155	30	29	28	27	27	26	25	24	24	23	22	22	21	20	20
160	31	30	29	28	27	27	26	25	24	24	23	22	22	21	21
165	32	31	30	29	28	27	27	26	25	24	24	23	22	22	21
170	33	32	31	30	29	28	27	27	26	25	24	24	23	22	22
175	34	33	32	31	30	29	28	27	27	26	25	24	24	23	22
180	35	34	33	32	31	30	29	28	27	27	26	25	24	24	23
185	36	35	34	33	32	31	30	29	28	27	27	26	25	24	24
190	37	36	35	34	33	32	31	30	29	28	27	26	26	25	24
195	38	37	36	35	33	32	31	31	30	29	28	27	26	26	25
200	39	38	37	35	34	33	32	31	30	30	29	28	27	26	26
205	40	39	37	36	35	34	33	32	31	30	29	29	28	27	26
210	41	40	38	37	36	35	34	33	32	31	30	29	28	28	27
215	42	41	39	38	37	36	35	34	33	32	31	30	29	28	28
220	43	42	40	39	38	37	36	34	33	32	32	31	30	29	28
225	44	43	41	40	39	37	36	35	34	33	32	31	31	30	29
230	45	43	42	41	39	38	37	36	35	34	33	32	31	30	30
235	46	44	43	42	40	39	38	37	36	35	34	33	32	31	30
240	47	45	44	43	41	40	39	38	36	35	34	33	33	32	31
245	48	46	45	43	42	41	40	38	37	36	35	34	33	32	31
250	49	47	46	44	43	42	40	39	38	37	36	35	34	33	32

How To Determine BMI

Height (feet & inches)

Weight (pounds)	5'0"	5'1"	5'2"	5'3"	5'4"	5'5"	5'6"	5'7"	5'8"	5'9"	5'10"	5'11"	6'0"	6'1"	6'2"	6'3"	6'4"
255	50	48	47	45	44	42	41	40	39	38	37	36	35	34	33	32	31
260	51	49	48	46	45	43	42	41	40	38	37	36	35	34	33	32	32
265	52	50	48	47	45	44	43	42	40	39	38	37	36	35	34	33	32
270	53	51	49	48	46	45	44	42	41	40	39	38	37	36	35	34	33
275	54	52	50	49	47	46	44	43	42	41	39	38	37	36	35	34	33
280	55	53	51	50	48	47	45	44	43	41	40	39	38	37	36	35	34
285	56	54	52	50	49	47	46	45	43	42	41	40	39	38	37	36	35
290	57	55	53	51	50	48	47	45	44	43	42	40	39	38	37	36	35
295	58	56	54	52	51	49	48	46	45	44	42	41	40	39	38	37	36
300	59	57	55	53	51	50	48	47	46	44	43	42	41	40	39	37	37
305	60	58	56	54	52	51	49	48	46	45	44	43	41	40	39	38	37
310	61	59	57	55	53	52	50	49	47	46	44	43	42	41	40	39	38
315	62	60	58	56	54	52	51	49	48	47	45	44	43	42	40	39	38
320	62	60	59	57	55	53	52	50	49	47	46	45	43	42	41	40	39
325	63	61	59	58	56	54	52	51	49	48	47	45	44	43	42	41	40
330	64	62	60	58	57	55	53	52	50	49	47	46	45	44	42	41	40
335	65	63	61	59	58	56	54	52	51	49	48	47	45	44	43	42	41
340	66	64	62	60	58	57	55	53	52	50	49	47	46	45	44	42	41
345	67	65	63	61	59	57	56	54	52	51	50	48	47	46	44	43	42
350	68	66	64	62	60	58	56	55	53	52	50	49	47	46	45	44	43
355	69	67	65	63	61	59	57	56	54	52	51	50	48	47	46	44	43
360	70	68	66	64	62	60	58	56	55	53	52	50	49	47	46	45	44
365	71	69	67	65	63	61	59	57	55	54	52	51	50	48	47	46	44
370	72	70	68	66	64	62	60	58	56	55	53	52	50	49	48	46	45
375	73	71	69	66	64	62	61	59	57	55	54	52	51	49	48	47	46
380	74	72	70	67	65	63	61	60	58	56	55	53	52	50	49	47	46
385	75	73	70	68	66	64	62	60	59	57	55	54	52	51	49	48	47
390	76	74	71	69	67	65	63	61	59	58	56	54	53	51	50	49	47
395	77	75	72	70	68	66	64	62	60	58	57	55	54	52	51	49	48
400	78	76	73	71	69	67	65	63	61	59	57	56	54	53	51	50	49

Factors associated with increased health risk: Your Realtor is right.

Your Realtor will relate the value of your property to three factors: location, location, location. With obesity, too, the location of fat is critical in determining health risk.

Obesity around the waist creates what obesity researchers call an apple shape. Obesity around the hips or thighs creates what researchers call a pear shape. (This shows that obesity researchers are always thinking of ways of introducing fruit into their daily lives.)

An apple shape causes more health risks than a pear shape. Those illnesses and conditions may affect you now and can increasingly affect you as you get older.

REMEMBER:
If you're shaped like a pear,
you'll need less Medicare!

Men tend to store more of their fat around the waist and in the abdominal cavity; as a result, men tend to be more apple-shaped and thus more at risk. So although women in general tend to be more concerned about their weight, men typically are at greater risk from their obesity.

What sort of fruit are you?

Although you can probably tell your shape by looking in a mirror, there is a simple formula for calculating your shape and its associated risks. It's called the *waist-to-hip ratio (WHR)*. It's calculated like this:

waist circumference (inches) divided by
hip circumference (inches)

To calculate the waist-to-hip ratio, you will need:
1. A tape measure
2. Your calculator
3. Your waist and your hips

A waist-to-hip ratio greater than 1.0 in men or 0.85 in women is associated with health risks.

An alternative way of calculating your waist-to-hip ratio is provided in the figure on page 12. Determine your waist circumference and mark the appropriate point on the waist circumference line. Determine your hip circumference and mark that point on the hip circumference line. Draw a line connecting the points on the waist and hip circumference lines. The point at which that line crosses the WHR line determines your waist-to-hip ratio.

It is also important to note that *the health risks associated with a high Body Mass Index are separate from those risks associated with a high waist-to-hip ratio. If you have a high BMI and a high waist-to-hip ratio, your risks are doubled.*

DID YOU KNOW?
The health risk calculation
of the waist-to-hip ratio
was devised by someone you know.
This person's identity is revealed
at the bottom of page 11.

Sample Waist-to-Hip Ratio Calculation

A man measures his waist and finds that it is 40 inches. He measures his hips (putting the tape measure around the largest part of his buttocks) and finds that this measurement is 36 inches.

His waist-to-hip ratio (WHR) is therefore 40 divided by 36. This gives him a WHR of 1.11.

Can an apple become a pear?

The distribution of your weight is determined by the location of your fat cells. Unfortunately, there isn't much you can do to change the distribution of your fat cells. For example, you cannot target fat cells by exercising one part of the body more than another; "spot reduction" is not possible. Such exercises will tone that part of the body but will not selectively reduce fat cell size or number. *The only effective way to cut back your health risks is to lose weight overall.*

Obesity and disease

There is continued debate about whether obesity is a disease in its own right. Obesity is certainly a chronic condition with associated medical risks. Some argue that obesity is more of a behavioral disorder than a medical one. But this is really a debate about the definition of the term *disease* that should not concern you unless you are a medical practitioner, philosopher, or lawmaker.

Answer: The calculation was developed by Ahmed H. Kissebah, M.D., Ph.D., scientific advisor to TOPS.

The major common diseases associated with obesity are:

- *Diabetes mellitus*—a disorder of carbohydrate metabolism that results in inadequate production and use of insulin.
- *Hypertension (high blood pressure)*—increased pressure on arteries that can result in degenerative damage to heart and kidneys.
- *Coronary artery disease*—a condition that reduces blood flow through the coronary arteries to the heart muscle.
- *Stroke*—a loss of sensation or voluntary movement caused by a rupture or an obstruction of an artery to the brain.
- *Cancer (especially of the breast, womb, prostate, and colon)*—a tumor of unlimited growth potential that invades other parts of the body.
- *Arthritis*—a condition in which cartilage and bone are worn down in various joints, resulting in pain.
- *Gall bladder disease*—an irritation of the gall bladder caused by deposits in the gall bladder sac and its ducts.

Remember that if you have a family history of these diseases, your risk is further increased.

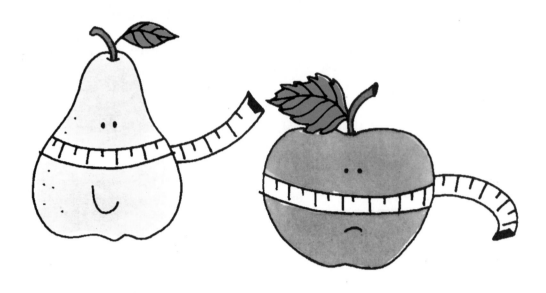

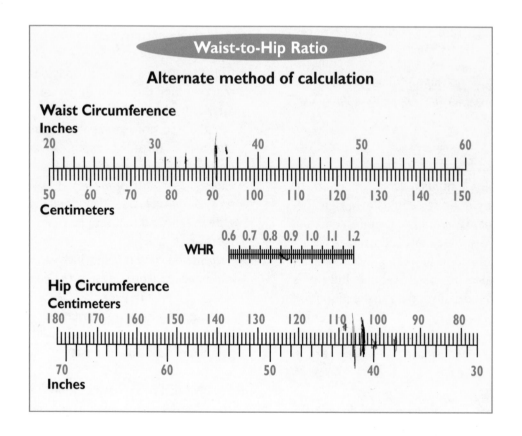

Waist-to-Hip Ratio

Alternate method of calculation

Waist Circumference
Inches

| 20 | 30 | 40 | 50 | 60 |

| 50 | 60 | 70 | 80 | 90 | 100 | 110 | 120 | 130 | 140 | 150 |

Centimeters

0.6 0.7 0.8 0.9 1.0 1.1 1.2

WHR

Hip Circumference
Centimeters

| 180 | 170 | 160 | 150 | 140 | 130 | 120 | 110 | 100 | 90 | 80 |

| 70 | 60 | 50 | 40 | 30 |

Inches

What causes obesity?

The answer is not as obvious as you may think.

You may see fat as a prison cell that traps you and restricts your freedom. Understanding another kind of cell—the fat cell—can be the key to successful treatment of your obesity.

What are fat cells?

Fat is a living organ made up of units called fat cells. These cells are like storage containers. Various factors influence the size, number, and location of fat cells. Nutrition obviously influences the size and number of your fat cells. Hormones also influence fat cell size, number, and location. Female hormones such as estrogen can cause an increase in fat cells in hips and thighs. Lack of female hormones can result in more fat cells around the waist. Male hormones such as testosterone can increase fat cells around the waist and between internal organs.

These hormonal influences help to explain why fat cell changes appear at certain times of life. During adolescence and pregnancy, when estrogen levels are at their highest, women frequently experience an increase in fat around the hips and thighs. When female hormones decline in menopause, fat around the waist may increase. In middle-aged men, male hormones promote an increase in fat around the waist.

How does liposuction work?

Liposuction is a surgical procedure in which fat cells are literally suctioned out of selected areas of the body. This procedure is performed through small holes in the skin. Its benefits can be temporary.

Although some fat cells may be removed from an area, it is possible that other cells left behind will grow to replace the suctioned ones. It is also possible that fat globules released from destroyed fat cells might seep into the bloodstream, blocking the blood supply to another part of the body. Scarring, bruising, and infection can also occur.

Do we need fat cells?

Fat cells are the most efficient form of energy storage. We need energy all the time to function efficiently, so having an effective energy storage system is important. As with everything else in life, however, there is a need for balance. Too little energy supply will make you tired and inefficient, but carrying around too many energy stores will do the same. There is no need to carry a power plant around with you when a few batteries are quite sufficient. It's all about balance!

Energy balance

There are two sides to the energy scale: energy intake and energy expenditure.

Energy intake
Your energy intake is determined solely by the amount and type of food you eat. Your body converts food into energy, which is calculated in units called calories.

In terms of energy, all calories count the same, regardless of their source. In other words, calories are calories whether they come from fruit, meat, or candy. (However, different foods do have different nutritional values beyond their caloric value, so not all foods are the same.)

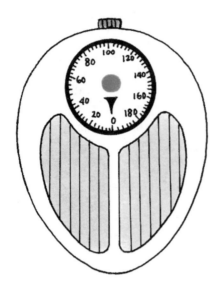

Certain types of food provide more calories than others. One gram of fat provides 9 calories, more than twice the amount provided by a gram of carbohydrate or protein.

Energy expenditure (see figure on page 15)
Your body constantly uses energy for essential life processes. For example, your heart pumps blood, your digestive system absorbs food, and your skeletal muscles move you around.

You can increase your energy expenditure by increasing muscle mass (getting more fit) and/or moving your skeletal muscles more (exercising).

• When your energy intake and expenditure are in balance, your body weight will be maintained.

• When your energy intake is greater than your expenditure, energy is stored as fat, and you will gain weight.

This energy balance is delicate. Small variations in food intake or energy expenditure will, over time, result in significant changes.

For example, imagine a thirty-year-old woman who weighs 150 pounds. On average, she eats 2,000 calories a day but expends only 1,900. Each week she stores 700 calories (100 calories each day for seven days). In the course of a year, she stores 36,400 extra calories (700 calories x fifty-two weeks). There are approximately 3,500 calories in a pound, so she would gain about 10 pounds per year. By the time she is forty, she will weigh 250 pounds!

Weight "creep" is the way most people gain their weight. Small increases in intake and/or small decreases in expenditure result in energy imbalances. Although these imbalances may be small, if they occur day after day, year after year, they will add significant weight.

DID YOU KNOW?
The brain contains centers
that influence your energy intake
(both the amount and type
of food you eat) and
energy expenditure (both muscle tone
and degree of activity).
Fat cells send chemical signals,
in the form of hormones
such as leptin, that tell the brain
how much fat is stored.

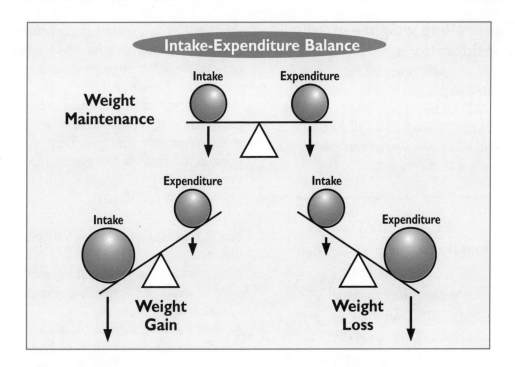

Intake-Expenditure Balance

Weight Maintenance — Intake — Expenditure

Expenditure — Intake — **Weight Gain**

Intake — Expenditure — **Weight Loss**

Is it all in my genes?

It is assumed that all bodily systems are influenced by genetics, and the energy balance mechanism is no exception. We know, for example, that adoptees' weights are strongly related to the weights of their biological parents but not their adoptive ones.

Yet although there is bound to be a genetic component to obesity, the key questions are *How much of the problem is due to genetics?* and *What, if anything, can be done for those with a strong genetic predisposition to obesity?*

It is estimated that while genetics play a large part (about 25 to 40 percent) in the development of obesity, environment plays an even bigger role (about 60 to 75 percent).

There is no way to change your genes. Life is not fair. Some people have genetic dispositions that allow them to eat almost anything in any amount and never gain weight, while others seem to gain weight by merely looking at food. *Regardless of your genetic predisposition, however, there are always things you can do that will help your problem.*

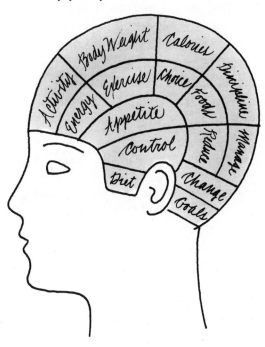

Controlling weight—medical considerations

Losing weight requires *action*. You will not lose weight just because you want to. You will not lose weight just by thinking about how to do it. *You will only lose weight when your energy expenditure exceeds your energy intake.*

ARE YOU READY. . .

. . . to make changes in eating and activity patterns?

. . . to meet the emotional demands of losing weight and keeping it off?

. . . to seek and utilize appropriate family and group support?

. . . to make weight management a priority in your life?

Setting an initial goal

You need to consider many factors when setting your weight goals, and these will be discussed in more detail in the following sections. As far as your health is concerned, you need to be aware of the following information.

Health improvements become apparent with the loss of 5 to 15 percent of body weight. For example, a woman weighing 200 pounds would get real health benefits by reducing her weight by 10 to 30 pounds. Such health improvements occur when BMI drops 2 units.

It is important to set an initial goal that will enable you to get some of these health benefits. Once you have achieved this initial level, it is more important to go on a maintenance regime to keep this new weight before attempting further weight loss. A realistic weight goal should, therefore, be individualized. It is the weight that you can achieve and, more importantly, maintain. There is no point in reducing your weight to a level that cannot be maintained by your physiology or your lifestyle.

Health benefits that come with weight loss include:
• Decreased blood sugar and less need for medications in those suffering from diabetes
• Decreased blood pressure and less need for medications in those with hypertension
• Decreased levels of "bad fats" and cholesterol
• Improved quality of life and improved self-esteem

The role of your physician

A physician can evaluate your obesity, monitor and treat any health complications, and provide expertise and support during a lifelong process. For these reasons, working closely with a physician is a central part of TOPS' philosophy.

Ideally, physicians help TOPS members by:
• Assessing health status, including obesity
• Determining readiness for weight loss
• Helping set reasonable and realistic weight goals
• Providing strategies to reduce weight or at least prevent further weight gain
• Referring TOPS members to other qualified weight-management professionals

The health assessment

Your health assessment should include:

- Accurate measures of height and weight
- Calculations of obesity and health risk using BMI and WHR
- Measures of vital signs, including blood pressure
- Blood tests to determine cholesterol and other blood fats
- Tests for the presence of other obesity-related illnesses, especially when you have symptoms and/or a family history of a particular condition
- Assessment of unhealthy lifestyle behaviors, especially those contributing to weight gain
- Assessment and possible screening for other medical conditions

PRACTICAL TIP:

If you have not had an assessment like the one described above, make an appointment with a physician now!

Your physician will also be able to determine your readiness to begin a program. For example, you may need to limit a particular exercise or increase a certain type of food (e.g., fiber) or nutritional supplement (e.g., vitamins or minerals). Also, certain conditions (such as pregnancy or gall bladder disease) make nutrition restriction inadvisable.

If, for some reason, your physician does not believe it is appropriate for you to begin a weight-reduction program immediately, work to develop a plan for leading the healthiest possible lifestyle. This should include a plan for *not gaining weight*.

A physician will also set you on your course by providing nutritional, fitness, and lifestyle guidelines. However, nutrition, exercise, and lifestyle change are all sciences in their own right, and your physician may enlist the aid of other professionals to help you in these areas.

PRACTICAL TIP:

If you feel you need more help in these areas than your physician is able or willing to give, ask for a referral to the appropriate health professional.

The role of the nutritionist

A nutritionist can provide basic information about nutrition, diet, and food choices. A nutritionist can take into account your usual diet, food preferences, eating habits, cooking techniques, and general lifestyle. From these, the nutritionist will devise a program to help you make better food choices by decreasing fat, sodium, and sugar intake and by adopting better eating habits in general.

The role of the physical fitness expert

The qualified exercise professional can inform you about the types, mechanics, and benefits of various exercises. This expert can also evaluate your fitness and customize an effective exercise program that takes into account your initial fitness level, age, gender, and lifestyle.

The role of the health behavior/lifestyle counselor

This trained professional can provide basic knowledge on how lifestyle influences health and weight. Besides assessing your current habits, this counselor can teach behavior change techniques (e.g., motivation, self-management, and habit change) that are crucial for successful application of knowledge supplied by the other health professionals.

Each of these professionals has a role to play, but you have the ultimate responsibility of keeping track of your progress.

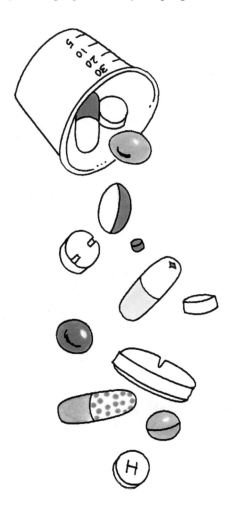

What about drugs?

There has been a lot of talk about anti-obesity drugs. Some of this is hype from nonprofessionals trying to market unproven products. Serious medications take years of development and must be rigorously tested before being brought to market. You should be suspicious of any sort of "pill" that has not received appropriate scientific and governmental support.

An ideal anti-obesity drug would:
• Reduce weight
• Maintain weight reduction
• Aid attempts to make lifestyle changes
• Produce selective loss of fat while sparing lean body mass
• Be safe, with minimal side effects and little potential for abuse

The drugs currently approved by the U.S. Food and Drug Administration (FDA) are appetite suppressants; they affect the brain centers that regulate food intake. Brain centers use certain chemicals—adrenaline and serotonin—to communicate with each other. These communicators determine when to eat and when to stop. Approved drugs for appetite control act like these chemicals to influence the food intake centers.

As much as we would like to believe that there is a magic bullet, no drugs will magically cure your obesity. Drugs do not remove the need for you to take responsibility for your health behaviors.

It is TOPS' policy not to encourage the use of drugs to achieve weight loss, because currently available drugs are not highly effective and could produce serious side effects. TOPS does, however, have an open mind about new discoveries in this field and hopes that new drug products that are effective and safe will be developed.

A word of caution

FDA-approved clinical trials have only tested currently available drugs for short-term use. These data do not include information on what happens to someone taking these pills for more than a year. Also, the weight losses achieved by people in clinical trials with these drugs are fairly modest. In addition, all drugs have side effects and cannot be used by some people.

Common side effects of some adrenaline-like drugs include hypertension, increased heart rate, restlessness, insomnia/fatigue, blurred vision, dry mouth, and constipation or diarrhea. Common side effects of some serotonin-like drugs include memory impairment, loss of coordination, fatigue or drowsiness, depression, pulmonary hypertension, and constipation or diarrhea.

As with many drugs, most side effects are experienced in the first few days of taking these anti-obesity medications and tend to moderate after continued use. Note, too, that side effects can be additive, especially when one is taking combinations of these drugs. Furthermore, the drugs should not be used if the person has renal (kidney) or liver disease, severe hypertension, heart failure, or pulmonary hypertension.

These drugs also should not be used if the person is pregnant or lactating; is using antidepressant or migraine medications; or has a history of substance abuse.

Are any new drugs available?

Other drugs are currently in development. We can only guess at how effective they might be and what their side effects may be.

Some of these new drugs work on the same brain chemicals as those drugs already approved by the FDA. Others work on different parts of the fat-control system. Some inhibit the production of pancreatic enzymes which break down fat and, thus, prevent absorption of fat from the gut into the bloodstream. When these are taken with food containing fat, less of the eaten fat is absorbed and the un-digested fat is excreted.

Other drugs are similar to natural hor-mones made by the body. Research sug-gests that fat tissue can produce a hor-mone thought to be the chemical messen-ger that informs the brain about the body's energy stores. Deficiency of, or insensitivity to these hormones is thought to be a cause of obesity. In this respect, these drugs represent a new generation of medication directed toward the cause of obesity. Their effectiveness and safety are currently being researched.

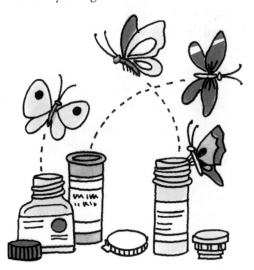

Cut it out?! The surgical options

Surgery is sometimes recommended for extremely obese individuals (those with a BMI of 40 or more) and particularly for those who have serious medical conditions such as difficult-to-control diabetes, hypertension, or disabling arthritis.

The goal of surgery is to limit food intake, digestion, and absorption. As with every other form of treatment, however, surgery is an aid and not an alternative to the usual weight-management strategies of a sensible diet and exercise regimen along with other healthy lifestyle changes.

Types of surgical procedures

Two types of surgery are currently used. In *modified gastric bypass*, the upper part of the stomach is connected directly to the lower gut. The person therefore cannot consume a large meal. This also means that food bypasses the stomach and is not fully digested. Undigested food is passed out with the stool. In *stomach banding*, plastic bands reduce the size of the stomach, forcing the individual to eat only small amounts.

Although significant weight loss can be achieved through surgery, there are potential complications. Wound infections and gall bladder disease are common. Leakage from the surgical site may also occur. In addition, the procedure can lead to nutritional and vitamin deficiencies and gut ulceration.

These surgical procedures should only be considered in severe or life-threatening cases. Such treatment is expensive and requires the assistance of experienced health care teams as well as a lifetime of follow-up with a surgeon.

Keeping your program going

Continuing your program after the first phase of weight loss is not easy, and the Lifestyle chapter of this guide includes tips designed to help keep your motivation going. There are, however, medical factors that influence your progress after you have lost some weight.

Plateaus, backsliding, and yo-yoing

Plateaus do not need to be the beginning of an uphill struggle. After the initial weight loss, it is common to experience a plateau or some weight regain, even if you stick to your weight-reduction program. One reason is that salt and water are rapidly depleted during the early phases of weight reduction. Once your body adjusts to the new regimen, some of this salt and water are replaced, giving the appearance of weight regain. As the levels of salt and water balance out, this type of plateau does not re-occur.

A second type of plateau is more serious and occurs in those who do not exercise. If you merely restrict your caloric intake without adding exercise, your metabolism slows down. If you only restrict your diet, especially if you take in a very low number of calories, your body considers itself to be in starvation mode and starts cutting back on some of its functions to conserve energy. This slows your metabolism, which is the last thing you want to do. Without exercise or activity to fire it up, your metabolism stays sluggish. Weight loss is a function of calories burned. The fewer calories you burn, the less weight you are going to lose.

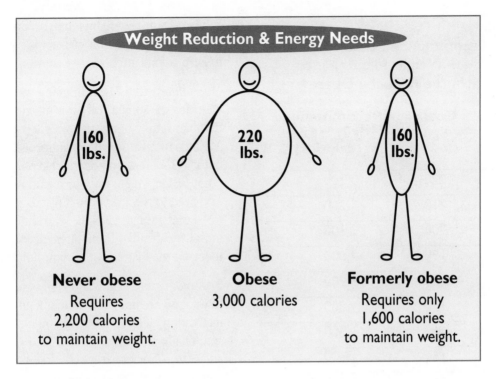

Weight Reduction & Energy Needs

Never obese
Requires
2,200 calories
to maintain weight.

Obese
3,000 calories

Formerly obese
Requires only
1,600 calories
to maintain weight.

PRACTICAL TIP:
Avoid a very-low-calorie diet unless specifically instructed to follow one by a physician.

Many people suffer from the yo-yo dieting syndrome in which they constantly lose and regain weight. This can lead to negative feelings, poor self-esteem, and a sense of failure.

There are several reasons for your weight swinging in this fashion, but one of the most important reasons is that once you have been obese, your body requires fewer calories to *maintain* weight.

When an obese person reduces caloric intake to lose weight, energy expenditure is slowed to a much lower level than for a never-obese person of the same weight.

This reduction in energy expenditure is thought to be genetic and a cause of obesity.

For example, imagine an obese person weighing 220 pounds who eats 3,000 calories a day to maintain weight. After reducing weight to 160 pounds, that person requires only 1,600 calories per day to balance expenditure needs. By contrast, someone of the same weight who has never been obese and has not reduced weight requires 2,200 calories a day to match energy expenditure and maintain weight.

This example highlights the need to reduce your energy intake and keep your energy expenditure as high as possible through good nutritional choices, sensible exercise, and lifestyle changes.

To calculate the appropriate calorie intake level for weight maintenance, see the table on the next page.

Recommended Caloric Intake for Weight Maintenance in the Reduced Obese*

Goal weight (lbs.)	Recommended daily intake (calories)
220	2,300
210	2,200
200	2,100
190	2,000
180	1,900
170	1,800
160	1,700
150	1,500
140	1,400
130	1,300
120	1,200

* "Reduced obese" are those who have successfully reduced weight to goal (15 percent below initial weight).

Recommended intake takes into account the decreased caloric expenditure of the reduced obese state.

Biology and genetics are not the only causes of backsliding and yo-yoing. These often occur because people lose their focus and stop making good choices because of:

• *Complacency.* Once you have lost some weight, it is easy to get complacent and assume that you can stop paying attention to your exercise and nutrition behaviors.

While certain new habits may become almost automatic after a while, it is crucial to keep paying attention to behavior.

• *Dwindling enthusiasm.* In many ways, watching the weight roll off is much more fun than simply preventing weight regain. Maintenance can seem unglamorous, but it is the key component. There is no point losing weight only to regain it. You need to reward yourself just as much for successful maintenance as you do for initial weight loss. In maintenance you focus on the benefits of all your efforts.

• *Lost motivation.* Motivation ebbs and flows. You are not going to maintain full motivation all of the time, so you must continually remind yourself of your goals and reasons for losing weight. Use the motivational techniques described in the Lifestyle chapter to stay focused enough of the time to make a difference.

A study of people who were successful at maintaining behavior change found that the *degree of vigilance* was the most critical difference between those who were successful and those who were not. To maintain changes, you need to continue to pay attention to your choices and stay focused on your goals.

Now that you understand more about the medical aspects of obesity, in the following chapters we'll see how exercise, nutrition, and other factors contribute to the condition and its management.

A quiz on medical perspectives

1) What Body Mass Index is associated with increased disease risk?
2) What waist-to-hip ratio is associated with increased disease risk for a man? . . . for a woman?
3) What percentage (within a range) of obesity is caused by genetics?
4) Significant health improvements occur when you have lost what percent of body weight?
5) When you reach a goal weight of 180 pounds, what is the recommended daily intake of calories to maintain that weight?

Answers:
1) 30 units
2) Man: 1.0 and above / woman: 0.85 and above
3) 25 to 40 percent
4) 5 to 15 percent
5) 1,900 calories

NUTRITION AND FOOD CHOICES

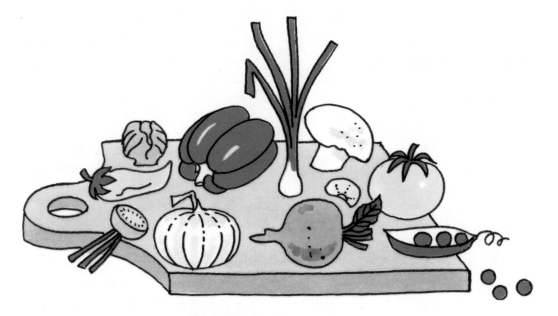

All the facts about nutrition will serve no purpose unless you are aware of your own eating patterns. The daily journal near the beginning of the 28-day guide later in this book provides a good format for recording your eating and exercise behavior. Make as many copies of that page as you will need to construct your own journal.

Now that you have learned about the energy balance equation and how it affects your weight, let's consider the first side of the equation, calorie intake. Obviously, it is critical that you know the basics of practical nutrition if you are going to evaluate claims made by food manufacturers, determine the best plan for you, and make healthy decisions.

In this section you will learn about:
- Basic nutrition facts
- Fat substitutes and low-calorie sweeteners
- Food labels and what they do and don't tell you
- The exchange system
- The food guide pyramid
- Vitamins and minerals
- Strategies for shopping, food preparation, portion control, snacking, eating out, and traveling

The dietary guidelines

The dietary guidelines are a set of recommendations on healthy nutrition for all North Americans over the age of two. To test your knowledge of these general recommendations, try this short quiz. Choose one answer from each set of three.

The guidelines state that you should:

1a) eat a variety of foods.
1b) eat only a few foods.
1c) choose just one thing and eat it for breakfast, lunch, and dinner.

2a) eat plenty of grains, vegetables, and fruit.
2b) have a diet low in grains, vegetables, and fruit.
2c) avoid grains, vegetables, and fruit like the plague.

3a) eat as much fat as you can get.
3b) never eat fat.
3c) eat a diet low in fat, saturated fat, and cholesterol.

4a) never have sugar.
4b) put sugar on everything you eat.
4c) eat a diet moderate in sugar.

5a) sprinkle large doses of salt on everything, including fruit.
5b) eat a diet moderate in salt and sodium.
5c) completely eliminate salt and sodium from your life.

6a) drink alcohol any place, anywhere, and anytime.
6b) never drink alcohol.
6c) use moderation if you drink alcohol.

Answers:
1a; 2a; 3c; 4c; 5b; 6c

The guidelines state that you should eat a variety of foods and choose a diet high in grains, vegetables, and fruit; low in fat; and moderate in sugar, salt, and sodium. Alcohol consumption should be moderate.

Basic facts about nutrition are presented below. These are all you need to know to implement healthy choices. You do not have to be a rocket scientist to choose a healthy diet.

Calories

Calories are units of energy that come from the metabolism of food in the body. All calories are the same, although different types of food generate different numbers of calories.

Carbohydrates provide 4 calories per gram.
Protein provides 4 calories per gram.
Fat provides 9 calories per gram.
Alcohol provides 7 calories per gram.

These are the calorie values of carbohydrates, proteins, and fats in their pure form. When you consume fat (e.g., oil, butter, or margarine), you are consuming only fat, and its calorie value is still 9 calories per gram. Carbohydrates and proteins, on the other hand, are usually present in foods like beans, pasta, and potatoes that also contain other nondigestible fibers and starches, so that 1 gram of these provides fewer than 2 calories.

You are probably saying to yourself, "Great! I know what alcohol is, but just what is a carbohydrate? A protein? A fat?"

Carbohydrates

There are two forms of carbohydrates. You know *simple carbohydrates* as sugar. These have only calories but no other nutritional value. *Complex carbohydrates*, on the other hand, are a better choice because they will be broken down by the body first and, due to fiber content, will provide fewer calories. They also contain vitamins, minerals, and other essential nutrients.

Examples of complex carbohydrates are fruits, vegetables, grains, cereals, and breads.

Proteins

Proteins contain the essential building blocks of life known as amino acids. Some of these amino acids are vital to body development and hormone production.

Foods that are rich in protein, particularly animal protein, also tend to be high in animal fat, so it is important to avoid excessive amounts of protein. The recommendation is that an adult who is not pregnant or lactating eat about 0.35 grams of protein per pound of body weight daily. Somebody weighing 200 pounds therefore requires about 70 grams of protein, generating 280 calories daily. This would represent about 20 percent of a 1,200-calorie diet.

Protein-rich foods include meats, fish, legumes, grains, and dairy products.

Fats

There are two types of fat: saturated and unsaturated.

Saturated fats are solid at room temperature and come mainly from animal products, although they are also found in chocolate, coconut, and palm oil.

An excess of saturated fats is not conducive to good health, especially since saturated fats help to increase levels of "bad" cholesterol in the blood.

One teaspoon contains 5 grams of fat, equal to 45 calories.

DID YOU KNOW?
Two-thirds of the calories in cheese come from saturated fat. Half of the calories in beef come from saturated fat. One-third of the calories in pork come from saturated fat. One-quarter of the calories in poultry and fish come from saturated fat.

Unsaturated fats are less dangerous to health than saturated fat. Unsaturated fats are either monounsaturated or polyunsaturated, depending on their chemical structure. Unlike saturated fats, these are soft or liquid at room temperature. They are found primarily in vegetable products like edible oils—safflower, sunflower, soybean, canola, corn, and olive oils—and also in fish.

Cholesterol

Cholesterol is a fat substance that circulates through the body, blood, and bile and is abundant in some body tissues, especially the nervous system. Cholesterol is normally produced by the liver, so it is not necessary to consume it.

Cholesterol is not the same as saturated fat. Foods that are high in saturated fat also tend to be high in cholesterol, but it is possible for a food to be low in saturated fat and high in cholesterol (e.g., shrimp).

Fiber

Fiber is essential to a healthy diet. It has two main health benefits: it decreases blood cholesterol and it helps food move through the gut. By enabling food to pass more quickly through the gut, fiber helps prevent bowel disease. In addition, a high-fiber food will make the person feel full and satisfied, thus helping to control food intake.

There are two types of fiber. Water-insoluble fiber (e.g., cellulose) is found in whole-wheat products and the skins of fruits and vegetables. Water-soluble fiber (e.g., pectin) is found in fruits, vegetables, beans, and oats.

The recommendation is to eat approximately 25 grams of fiber daily. To achieve this, try to include two fiber-rich foods at each meal. Breakfast is a particularly good time to get your fiber. Cereal, whole-wheat bread, bran, and fruit are all good sources of fiber.

Grams of Fiber in Various Foods

1 oz. wheat bran	11.3
$1/2$ cup raspberries	9.2
1 cup cooked broccoli	6.5
1 cup brown rice	4.5
1 pear	4.0
1 bran muffin	4.0
2 slices whole-wheat bread	3.2
apple (medium)	3.2
orange	2.8

It is also important to take enough fluid when you eat fiber-rich foods, since fiber absorbs fluid. If fluid is not present, the food will ferment, causing uncomfortable and potentially embarrassing gas.

Sodium

Your body requires sodium. Many people, however, consume far more than the body needs, and this can increase the risk of high blood pressure and kidney problems.

Even if you do not suffer from these problems, it is advisable to moderate sodium intake. Hypertension and kidney problems frequently appear later in life. Cutting back on sodium now will help reduce your risk of having these serious health problems later.

Most people will lower their blood pressure when they reduce sodium intake. Studies show that, within reason, lower blood pressure is related to improved health, so even if your blood pressure is normal, you can still benefit from reducing your salt intake.

A major source of sodium intake is processed foods—packaged, canned, and frozen goods. About 65 percent of sodium intake comes from these sources, while the remaining 35 percent comes from the salt shaker.

Maximum sodium intake should be less than 3,000 milligrams per day. Remember, one teaspoon of salt contains approximately 2,300 milligrams of sodium.

If you eat a lot of salty foods or add salt to your foods, it is important to change this habit. High intake of salt is an acquired behavior; you are not born with this preference. Once you have adjusted to a reduced sodium intake, food will be just as tasty. You will find it easy to *shake* the habit.

PRACTICAL TIP:
Taste the food before
you reach for the salt.

Alcohol

Some researchers suggest that moderate consumption of alcoholic beverages could be beneficial to health. Some of these benefits, however, can be achieved just as well through other means, like a low-fat diet, exercise, and a healthy lifestyle.

Remember, alcohol is a powerful drug that can impair your control and judgment. In addition, alcohol can be a big diet-buster for the following reasons:

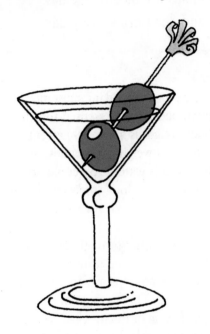

- Alcohol contains significant numbers of calories.
  - A 12-oz. regular beer has 150 calories.
  - A 12-oz. lite beer has 100 calories.
  - A 4-oz. glass of wine has 85 calories.
  - A 4-oz. Manhattan has 219 calories.

- Alcohol has no nutritional value other than the calories it provides. That is why alcohol is sometimes referred to as having "empty calories."

- Your willpower may dissolve in alcohol. Your perception, judgment, and control could deteriorate once you have too much of it.

- For many people, alcohol stimulates appetite.

PRACTICAL TIP:
Have no more than 200 calories in alcohol on any one day, and don't drink every day.

Water

Water is the most abundant substance in the human body and is essential for life. Your body weight is about 60 percent water, so if you weigh 150 pounds, 90 pounds of you is water! You could go many days without food (theoretically, at least) but only a few days without water.

The body loses water through digestion, breathing, sweating, and urination. If these losses are not replenished, the body gets dehydrated. The first sign of dehydration is the feeling of thirst, which begins when approximately 2 percent of your body water is not replenished. Drink water to avoid thirst, not just to quench it.

We recommend that a TOPS member drink eight 8-oz. glasses of water daily to meet essential body requirements. Drinks that contain caffeine, such as coffee, tea, and caffeinated sodas, are not as effective as water itself because they stimulate larger-than-normal water loss in the urine. In this case, you need to drink additional water to replace this water loss.

Drinking water regularly also has the advantage of making you feel full, thus decreasing hunger. As you will see in the section on managing high-risk situations, this makes drinking water a good first response in a tempting situation.

PRACTICAL TIP:
Keep a water bottle filled, and sip from it throughout the day.

Sugar

As discussed earlier, sugars are simple carbohydrates. They have no nutritional value besides providing calories. There are different forms. Fructose, found in fruits, and sucrose, found in refined sugar, have different chemical structures.

There are several reasons to be moderate in your intake of sugar. Sugar calories add up quickly. Like all calories, sugar calories contribute to your overall intake. A teaspoon of sugar has 16 calories. If you put one teaspoon of sugar in your cereal and two in your tea or coffee at breakfast, you have consumed 48 calories. Let's suppose that you have another cup of tea or coffee at mid-morning, one at lunch, one in mid-afternoon, one at dinner, and one after dinner. That's another five cups, and with two teaspoons of sugar in each you have added another ten teaspoons of sugar at the cost of 160 extra calories. Include breakfast and you have 208 calories from added sugar. And that does not include sugar from other sources, like the cereal itself, soft drinks, and other treats you might have during the day. Remember, an extra 208 calories every day for a year adds up to 75,920 calories, which is the equivalent of gaining 21 pounds!

Also bear in mind that many sugary foods are also high in fat. For instance, cakes and other baked goods are high in both sugar and fat.

Habitual intake of sugar can make blood-glucose levels unstable, particularly in an obese person. Blood glucose levels rise with the intake of sugar and then decline. During the decline, especially if it is rapid, one might feel physically uncomfortable, moody, agitated, lightheaded, and hungry. A fluctuating blood-glucose level is not good for mood or for weight-control efforts. It is best to keep your blood-glu-cose level on an even keel by eating small, frequent meals and minimizing sugar intake. This blood-glucose level phenome-non seems to prime some people to eat sugar. Once they have eaten some sugar, they find it difficult to stop.

Although sugar initially gives a quick fix of energy, in anything other than the short term, sugar actually *depletes* energy. A high intake of sugar will, in the end, make the person feel lethargic.

In the section on sugar substitutes, you will learn the best alternatives to sugar. Some sugar in moderation is fine, but one of the easiest ways of cutting back on overall calorie consumption is by limiting sugar use.

PRACTICAL TIP:
Use sugar substitutes at least
some of the time.

Caffeine

Excessive caffeine, like excessive sugar, can deplete energy. Although caffeine does give a jolt of energy immediately after consumption, it depletes energy in the long run. Caffeine can initially cause overarousal, so it is not a good choice for a person who is already stressed.

Caffeine is also addictive. Sixteen percent of people who drink four or more cups of coffee a day show signs of dependence. If the person becomes caffeine dependent, withdrawal symptoms will occur. Caffeine withdrawal symptoms, which usually last about 48 hours, consist mainly of fatigue, lethargy, and headache.

Caffeine is found in coffee, tea, chocolate, and some sodas. A cup of coffee contains about 100 milligrams of caffeine.

PRACTICAL TIP:
Limit your caffeine intake to
no more than 200 milligrams a day
(the amount found in
two cups of coffee).

Fat substitutes and low-calorie sweeteners

Can I have my cake and eat it, too?

In recent years, there has been much interest in the development of fat substi-tutes that attempt to reduce fat in foods while preserving their taste and appeal. There are three types of fat substitutes.

1. *Calorie-reduced substitutes that are digested by the body.* These are derived from carbohydrates which are modified to form a gel-like substance, giving

the taste characteristics of fats and oils. These substitutes are found in frozen desserts, spoonable and pourable salad dressings, sour cream type products, yogurt, sauces, gravies, and puddings.

2. *Calorie-free substitutes that are not digested by the body.* These are manufactured from edible oils such as soybean, corn, or cottonseed. The oils are converted into a chemical structure that prevents them from being digested and absorbed in the blood. They cannot, therefore, be used by the body to provide calories. This type of substitute is now used instead of regular oils in some brands of potato chips, corn and tortilla chips, cheese puffs, and crackers.

3. *Calorie-reduced substitutes for traditional foods.* These are products formulated with less than 1/2 gram of fat per serving. These low-fat versions of foods have been introduced in processed cheese, salad dressings, yogurt, frozen yogurt, frozen desserts, frozen dessert bars, and low-fat baked goods. Like the first type of calorie-reduced substitutes, these are digested by the body.

WARNING!
Fat substitutes do not make a food calorie-free.
These foods may not have fat in them (or may have very little fat), but they still have carbohydrates and proteins. A 1-oz. serving of regular potato chips has 150 calories; a 1-oz. serving of potato chips made with calorie-free fat substitute still provides 70 calories.

Neither do fat substitutes make a food healthy. Many of the fat-free foods are very high in sugar, which, as you have already seen, can create unstable blood-glucose levels and problems with mood, energy levels, and hunger.

Fat-free foods are acceptable as part of a balanced diet, allowing you to have something close to the original foods without adding fat.

PRACTICAL TIPS:
For cooking, stir-frying, or sauteing, use clear chicken broth, cooking wine, vermouth, vinegar, or water.
Use a low-fat cooking spray to coat pans and skillets.
For topping potatoes and vegetables, use fat-free ranch dressing, salsa, liquid butter-flavored products made from mixes, or fat-free squeeze margarine.

How sweet is it?
A look at sugar substitutes
You have already learned how important it is to moderate your intake of sugar. There are at least three reasons to watch your sugar intake. They are. . . well, you tell us. Answers appear below.

Given that moderate sugar intake is your goal and given also that you like sweet-tasting foods, how acceptable are the sugar substitutes?

Answers:
Sugar can increase hunger, add calories, and deplete energy.

Sugar substitutes are intended to provide sweet taste without the calories that go with sugar. Some of these sweeteners have no calories. Those approved by the FDA include saccharin, aspartame, acesulfame-K, and sucralose. Some low-calorie sweeteners are natural sugars, including fructose, sorbitol, xylitol, and mannitol. These yield 4 calories per gram—the same as sugar—but because their sweetening power is three times greater than sugar, one can use less of them (at least in theory!)

Some sweeteners work best in cold foods; others work well in cooking and baking. For best results, use a recipe that specifies a low-calorie sweetener rather than replacing the sugar in a regular recipe.

On page 34 are some basic guidelines for choosing and using various sweeteners.

Calories in Some Foods Containing Sugar Substitutes

Sugar-free pudding	80 calories per 1/2 cup
Sugar-free, low-fat yogurt	80 calories per 1/2 cup
Regular stick of gum	7 calories
Sugar-free stick of gum	5 calories
Diet soda	<1 calorie
Sugar-free gelatin	<1 calorie

Take advantage of the sweet taste of foods and drinks made with low-calorie sweeteners, but remember that these foods may still have calories. Don't be lulled into a false sense of security that somehow these calories don't count as part of your overall intake.

The best advice is to limit the amount of sweets that you eat. Replace your sweet snacks with healthy foods like fruits and vegetables.

Reduce the amount of sugar in a recipe by one-third. You won't alter the taste much, and the finished product will still maintain color and tenderness.

Remember, too, that although the FDA has approved these sugar substitutes as safe when used in limited quantities, there is still some controversy about potential health risks for some individuals. You need to make your own judgment about the kind and level of your usage of these products, consulting with a physician or qualified health professional if necessary.

PRACTICAL TIP:
Use calorie-free, sugar-free syrup on your next pancake. An average serving of regular syrup has 300 calories.

Food labels
Recent changes in food labeling make it easier to track the important ingredients in foods. However, use care when reading everything from serving sizes, saturated fat, and fiber content to daily recommended allowances.

Sweetener Guide

Product	Major sweetening agent	Sweetness compared to sugar	Suggested uses
EQUAL (packets or tablets)	Aspartame	1 packet = 2 tsp. sugar 1 tablet = 1 tsp. sugar	Table use: Add to cold/hot foods after cooking. Equal will not withstand high temperatures over the long term.
NUTRASWEET (spoonful)	Aspartame	1 tsp. = 1 tsp. sugar	Table use: Add to cold or non-baked dishes.
SPRINKLE SWEET (packets)	Saccharin	1 packet = 2 tsp. sugar	Baking, cooking, and table use. Use toward the end of the cooking process; can get bitter if exposed to heat over a long period.
SUGAR TWIN (regular & brown sugar replacements: powder & packets)	Saccharin	1 tsp. = 1 tsp. sugar 1 cup = 1 cup sugar 1 packet = 2 tsp. sugar	Baking, cooking, and table use. Use toward the end of the cooking process; can get bitter if exposed to heat over a long period.
SWEET 10 (liquid)	Saccharin	10 drops = 1 tsp. sugar 2 Tbsp. = 1 cup sugar 1 packet = 2 tsp. sugar	Cooking and table use. Use toward the end of the cooking process; can get bitter if exposed to heat over a long period.
SWEET 'N LOW (regular & brown sugar replacement: powder & packets)	Saccharin	1 tsp. = $1/4$ cup sugar 1 packet = 2 tsp. sugar	Cooking and table use. Use toward the end of the cooking process; can get bitter if exposed to heat over a long period.
SWEET ONE (packets)	Acesulfame-K	1 packet = 2 tsp. sugar 6 packets = $1/2$ cup sugar	Table use and cooking.
FRUCTOSE (powder & packets)	Fructose (sugar from fruit)	1 tsp. = 1 Tbsp. sugar 1 packet = 1 Tbsp. sugar	Cooking and table use. May taste sweeter in cold foods, so use sparingly.

Serving sizes

Serving sizes are now set by the FDA, not by the manufacturer. Standard serving sizes are based on the amount that the FDA considers people most often eat as a single serving. Unfortunately, some serving sizes have been set too small, others too large. For example, the serving size for poultry, fresh meat, and seafood is 3 oz. (cooked)—considerably less than what the average person usually eats.

The label can also list the "raw" or "cooked" values, which leaves *you* cooked because it is not always possible to compare the two!

EXCHANGE SYSTEM WARNING!
The serving size listed on the food label often does not correspond to a serving in the exchange system. For example, the food label describes a single serving of bread as *two* slices because that is considered the most common serving eaten. A serving of bread in the exchange system is *one* slice. (See "Exchanges for common foods" in the Appendix.)

Saturated fat

You have already learned about the health risks of consuming too much saturated fat. The food label now has to indicate how many of the fat grams are saturated fat.

Fiber

The label lists grams of fiber per serving. This will make it easier for you to reach your target of at least 25 grams of fiber daily.

Daily allowance

The label indicates the percentage of your recommended daily allowance for each nutrient. However, the allowance is based on a daily intake of 2,000 calories. Your intake level for weight management is going to be less than this. Remember, you must be very careful in using the daily allowance on labels as a guide for your planned diet.

Also, be aware that if a food provides 20 percent or more of the daily allowance (again calculated on the basis of a 2,000-calorie diet), then it's "high" in that nutrient. If a food provides 5 percent or less, it is considered "low" in this nutrient.

The values for sugars are included under total carbohydrates. For a weight-control program, however, you need to limit sugar consumption to 50 grams or less. Sugars that are naturally present in the food, as well as added sugar, are lumped together in the same category; so foods like yogurt, cereal with fruit, milk, and fruit juices will appear high in sugar because they contain natural sugar.

Listing of ingredients

Ingredients are listed on the label in order by their weight. The item which weighs the most is listed first, and the rest are listed in descending order.

This means that you know the relative weight but not how much of a certain ingredient is in a food. For example, a fruit juice label might read: *Water, apples, corn syrup.* You know that there is more water than apples, but you do not know how much more.

Nutrient content claims: What *free, low, lean,* and other terms mean

New regulations have been imposed on nutrient claims. This has eliminated many misleading claims, but not all of them.

Previously, the word *free* on a food label was almost meaningless. Now, if a food is labeled *sugar free* or *fat free,* it means that the food contains none of that nutrient or only a trace of it.

WARNING!

Watch out for the phrase *cholesterol free* **food.**
The presence of the word *food* could mean that the product never had any cholesterol to begin with! So much for the bananas that carried a "no cholesterol" label. Now, only when a company takes cholesterol out of a food can it use the term *cholesterol free.*

Labels that advertise a nutrient as *low-calorie* indicate that it can be eaten regularly without exceeding the (2,000-calorie-per-day) dietary guidelines. *Low fat* indi-

cates foods with 3 grams or less of fat per serving. *Low saturated fat* indicates foods with less than 1 gram of saturated fat per serving. *Low sodium* indicates food with 140 milligrams or less of sodium per serving.

So, now you can purchase a low-fat frozen dinner completely safe in the knowledge that it has less than 3 grams of fat, right? Well, you might feel safe, but you would be wrong! *The 3-grams-of-fat rule applies only to individual foods.*

Nutrition Facts
Serving Size 1/2 cup (114g)
Servings Per Container: 4

Amount Per Serving

Calories 91	Calories From Fat 27

%Daily Value *

Total Fat 3g	5%
Saturated Fat 0g	0%
Cholesterol 0mg	0%
Sodium 300mg	13%
Total Carbohydrate 13g	4%
Dietary Fiber 3g	12%
Sugars 3g	
Protein 3g	

Vitamin A	80%	Vitamin C	2%
Calcium	4%	Iron	4%

* Percent Daily Values based on a 2,000 calorie diet. Your daily values may be higher or lower depending on your calorie needs.

	Calories	1,500	2,000
Total Fat	Less than	45g	65g
Sat Fat	Less than	15g	20g
Cholesterol	Less than	300mg	300mg
Sodium	Less than	2,400mg	2,400mg
Total Carbohydrate		225g	300g
Fiber		20g	25g

Calories per gram:

Fat 9 • Carbohydrates 4 • Protein 4

The term *lean* is used to describe the fat content of meat, poultry, or fish. *Lean* means less than 10 grams of fat in a 3½-oz. serving. If a product is *extra lean*, it has 5 grams or less of fat in a 3½-oz. serving.

Lean claims are only useful when they appear on fresh cuts of meat or poultry. The term *lean* was established to help people identify low-fat meats. Any food, however, can call itself *lean* if it has no more than 10 grams of fat, 4½ grams of saturated fat, and 95 milligrams of cholesterol. Many foods that satisfy those criteria would not be considered low-fat.

Other terms
Good source means that a serving of the food supplies 10 to 19 percent of the daily allowance for a particular nutrient, again based on a 2,000-calorie-per-day diet.

Reduced means that a serving of the food has been altered to contain 25 percent less of the nutrient than is present in the unaltered food.

Light means that the calories in a food have been reduced by at least a third of the regular food or that the fat content has been halved.

What the label does not tell you
There is certain information that the food label does not tell you.

Labels no longer list the level of B vitamins, such as thiamin, riboflavin, and niacin, unless the product has been fortified with them. The FDA believes that deficiencies of these vitamins are no longer a health concern in the U.S. and therefore does not require them to be listed.

Labels do not list fat content in children's food. In fact, baby and toddler food must *not* show information about calories from fat, because the FDA wants to prevent parents from wrongly assuming that their young children should restrict fat. Fat is an important nutrient during the first two years of life.

Also notice that restaurants are not required to provide nutrition information about the food they serve.

Why good things don't necessarily come in small packages

Any package smaller than 12 square inches does not have to provide nutrition information on the label. It does, however, have to provide an address or telephone number for consumers who wish to obtain this information. So the next time you are in a service station about to buy one of those tempting snacks, make sure you buy some paper, an envelope, and a stamp, too, so you can get the nutrition information in writing before you eat.

Food guides: How to plan a nutritionally healthy weight-management program

By now you have enough information about the basics of nutrition, foods, and nutrients as well as food labels. The next step is to learn how to make healthy food choices that help you begin and maintain a weight-control program. You need to learn about this process and also to practice it so frequently that it becomes part of your daily routine, like brushing your teeth before going to bed. To do this, you need to know the two main guides that can help you plan healthy eating: the exchange system and the food guide pyramid.

TOPS strongly recommends the exchange system to its members as the starting point of a weight-loss program. You will also learn how to use the food guide pyramid, which is a useful alternative for some people.

The exchange system shows how to select and quantify food choices. It gives you variety and flexibility in your meal planning while providing specific portion sizes.

The food guide pyramid is a visual method for making food choices. It is quick to use, but its disadvantage is the risk of overestimating portion sizes, which may jeopardize your weight-control efforts. The advice is to use the food guide pyramid only when you can reliably judge portion sizes.

Caloric intake goals

As discussed in Chapter 1, most experts agree that the personal skills and behaviors needed for weight loss are different from those needed to maintain weight after goal is reached. When your weight-loss goal has been determined and you are ready to begin this task, you should start a sensible weight-reduction program. The recommended daily caloric intake during this phase depends on your gender and BMI as follows:

> For a male with a BMI less than 30: 1,500 calories
> For a male with a BMI greater than 30: 1,800 calories
>
> For a female with a BMI less than 30: 1,200 calories
> For a female with a BMI greater than 30: 1,500 calories

In general, no one should eat fewer than 1,200 calories per day, regardless of gender or degree of overweight.

The benefits of a weight-reduction diet, particularly over the long term, will only be realized if the diet is accompanied by an exercise program, healthy lifestyle changes, and group support.

Once you have reached your goal and wish to maintain your new weight, you can adjust your caloric intake. To determine your recommended caloric intake during this phase, refer to the table on page 22. Again, success depends on keeping up your exercise program, lifestyle changes, and group support.

The exchange system
What is it?

As you have learned, calories are derived from three nutrient sources: carbohydrate, protein, and fat. Dietitians have divided all foods into six groups. Foods are grouped together because they contain similar proportions of these three nutrients.

The foods in each group are matched by their amounts of carbohydrate, protein, and fat, not by calories. The exchange portion is determined by each food's weight in grams. This is why it is possible to "exchange" one food on the list for another on the same list. Each group has the same weight of the three major nutrients in grams. The number of calories for one exchange is also provided.

Nutrient Content of One Exchange

Exchange group	Carbohydrate grams	Protein grams	Fat grams	Calories per exchange
STARCH/BREAD	15	3	0-1	80
FRUIT	15	0	0	60
MILK				
Nonfat	12	8	0-3	90
Low-fat	12	8	5	120
Whole	12	8	8	150
VEGETABLES	5	2	0	25
MEAT/MEAT SUBSTITUTES				
Very lean	0	7	0-1	35
Lean	0	7	3	55
Medium-fat	0	7	5	75
High-fat	0	7	8	100
FAT	0	0	5	45

Sample Exchange Lists

1,200-calorie diet	1,500-calorie diet	1,800-calorie diet
BREAKFAST		
1 milk exchange	1 milk exchange	1 milk exchange
1 starch/bread exchange	1 starch/bread exchange	1 starch/bread exchange
1 fruit exchange	1 fruit exchange	1 fruit exchange
1 meat exchange	1 meat exchange	1 meat exchange
1 fat exchange	1 fat exchange	1 fat exchange
free food	free food	free food
LUNCH		
1 starch/bread exchange	2 starch/bread exchanges	2 starch/bread exchanges
1 fruit exchange	1 fruit exchange	1 fruit exchange
2 meat exchanges	2 meat exchanges	2 meat exchanges
1 vegetable exchange	2 vegetable exchanges	2 vegetable exchanges
1 fat exchange	1 fat exchange	1 fat exchange
free food	free food	free food
DINNER		
2 starch/bread exchanges	2 starch/bread exchanges	2 starch/bread exchanges
1 fruit exchange	1 fruit exchange	1 fruit exchange
2 meat exchanges	2 meat exchanges	3 meat exchanges
1 vegetable exchange	2 vegetable exchanges	2 vegetable exchanges
1 fat exchange	1 fat exchange	2 fat exchanges
free food	free food	free food
SNACKS		
1 starch/bread exchange	1 starch/bread exchange	1 starch/bread exchange
1 milk exchange	1 milk exchange	1 milk exchange
free food	1 fruit exchange	2 fruit exchanges
	free food	1 fat exchange
		free food

The six exchange groups are starch/bread, meat, fruits, vegetables, milk, and fat. The table on page 39 provides the nutrients and calories in one exchange for each of the groups.

How can I use this exchange system?

To use the exchange system, all you need to know is the group to which a food belongs. Then fit that food into the exchange diet plan. Let's try it, using the sample exchange list for the 1,200-calorie diet.

A starch/bread exchange is a 1-oz. slice of white bread. Careful—not all slices are equal! A description of serving size or weight is necessary. A 1-oz. serving of bread can be exchanged for any of the following:

2 slices diet bread
$1/2$ English muffin
2-oz. waffle
$1^1/2$ cups puffed wheat cereal
$1/2$ cup sugar-frosted cereal
2 rice cakes (4" across)
$2/3$ cup cooked oatmeal

Our exchange list calls for one starch/bread exchange at breakfast. We could have:

$1^1/2$ cups puffed wheat cereal

We'll record this on a sample Daily Journal sheet on the next page. What would you choose? Write the answer in your journal (make a photocopy of page 136).

Other starchy foods are found in this bread group, including squash, pasta,

potatoes, and corn. Each $1/2$-cup serving of these provides the same amount of carbohydrate, protein, fat, and calories as one slice of bread.

Our exchange list advises one starch/bread exchange for lunch. We could have:

2 slices diet bread for a sandwich

What would you choose? Write the answer in your journal.

Our exchange list advises two starch/bread exchanges for dinner. We could have:

1 cup spaghetti

What would you choose? Write the answer in your journal.

Our exchange list allows one starch/bread exchange as a snack. We could have:

2 rice cakes

What would you choose? Write the answer in your journal.

Remember: Measure the serving size of a bread or starch portion. It is all too easy to decide that a single serving of cereal is the one that fits your bowl!

A fruit exchange is much easier to understand. It's just fruit! And all the calories come from the same nutrient: carbohydrates. One fruit exchange has 15 grams of carbohydrate and 60 calories.

Fruit servings need to be small; let's call them about the size of a tennis ball. An

THE DAILY JOURNAL

Keeping a daily journal is an important way to monitor your behavior and assess your progress. Use the format below and/or the TOPS exchange recorder to keep track of your own program or the 28-day program provided with this guide. Photocopy this page or order your reusable exchange recorder (item M-7) through your chapter (form L-15).

Date: _____   Daily intake goals: _____   Daily exercise expenditure goal: _____

Food Consumed:

Meal	Food/amount	Fat gm	Cals.
Breakfast	1 1/2 cups puffed wheat cereal	0-1	80
	2 Tbsp. raisins	0	60
	1 cup nonfat milk	0-3	90
	1/4 cup cottage cheese (4-5% fat)	5.5	77.5
Lunch	2 slices diet bread	0-1	80
	2 oz. lean roast beef	11	155
	1 frozen fruit bar	0	60
	4 black olives, large	2.5	23
Dinner	1 cup spaghetti	0-2	160
	2 oz. meatballs (made with ground round)	11	155
	1/2 cup spaghetti sauce (meatless)	0	50
	1 1/4 cups strawberries	0	60
Snacks	2 rice cakes	0-1	80
	1 cup plain yogurt, nonfat, sugar-free	0-3	90
TOTAL		30-41	1,220.5

Comments:

Exercise Done:

Exercise	Time	Time spent	Calories burned
Other activities			
TOTAL			

Comments:

apple should be approximately 2" in diameter. If you choose a larger piece of fruit, you will be eating two fruit exchanges and twice the calories.

Take caution with fruit juices. That 15 grams of carbohydrate, or one fruit exchange, limits you to 1/2 cup fruit juice. If you fill the glass with juice, you may have two or even three fruit exchanges. On a warm summer day, those exchanges and calories can mount quickly.

Examples of fruit exchanges include:

   1 small apple
   1/3 small cantaloupe
   1/2 cup fruit cocktail
   17 small grapes
   2 Tablespoons raisins
   1 1/4 cups strawberries
   1 1/4 cups watermelon cubes
   1/3 cup prune juice
   1/2 cup orange juice

Our exchange list calls for one fruit exchange at breakfast. We could now add:

   2 Tablespoons raisins

to the 1 1/2 cups of puffed wheat cereal we chose for our starch/bread exchange. What would you choose? Write the answer in your journal.

Our exchange list allows one fruit exchange at lunch. We could have:

   1 frozen fruit bar

along with the two slices of diet bread in our sandwich. What would you choose? Write the answer in your journal.

Our exchange list allows one fruit exchange at dinner. We could have:

   1 1/4 cups strawberries

in addition to the 1 cup spaghetti we chose for our starch/bread exchange. What would you choose? Write the answer in your journal.

Remember: One fruit exchange equals 1/2 cup of most canned fruits and juices.

The exchange system has one more group where we will find carbohydrates: the milk group. Surprisingly, milk has almost the same amount of carbohydrates as bread. An 8-oz. glass of milk has 12 grams of carbohydrate, and a slice of bread has 15 grams of carbohydrate. Protein and varying amounts of fat are also present.

You will want to stay with low-calorie choices. Remember, the higher the fat content of milk or yogurt, the higher the calories climb:

   8 oz. nonfat milk…90 calories (no fat)
   8 oz. reduced fat (2%) milk…120 calories
      (5 grams fat, equal to 1 pat butter)
   8 oz. whole milk…150 calories (8 grams
      fat, equal to 1.6 pats butter)

In the example above, carbohydrate and protein amounts remain the same. Only the fat content changes.

Examples of milk exchanges include:
   1 cup nonfat or low-fat milk
   1 cup plain yogurt, nonfat, sugar-free
   1/2 cup evaporated milk

Our exchange list calls for one milk exchange at breakfast. We could add:

1 cup nonfat milk

to our 2 Tablespoons raisins and 1½ cups puffed wheat cereal. What would you choose? Write the answer in your journal.

Our exchange list allows one milk exchange as a snack. We could have:

　1 cup plain yogurt, nonfat, sugar-free

What would you choose?
Write the answer in your journal.

Remember: One exchange from the milk group equals 8 fluid ounces. Pay attention to the fat content of your choices.

Foods in the meat and meat substitutes list contain both protein and fat—no carbohydrate. That's why cheese is found in this grouping rather than with the milk group. Cheese has no whey (the carbohydrate found in milk). Cheese is mainly protein and fat.

Most of the foods that belong in this group would be suitable in a sandwich: meat, cheese, peanut butter.

Again, fat levels will alter your calorie intake. Caution is necessary.

　1 turkey hot dog…100 calories
　1 fat-free turkey hot dog…35 calories
　1 oz. chipped beef…35 calories
　1 oz. corned beef…100 calories

Fat levels vary, so meats have been divided into subgroups of very lean, lean, medium-fat, and high-fat. Despite that variation, one ounce is one serving for all subgroups of meat.

Do not get confused when applying our diet exchange lists. A recommendation of two meat exchanges does *not* mean you should prepare two different meat entrees tonight! It describes a portion of 2 ounces.

Examples of one meat exchange include:

　1 oz. chicken or turkey
　1 oz. cheese
　¼ cup cottage cheese
　1 egg
　1 oz. tuna
　2 medium sardines
　1 oz. beef, pork, or veal

Our exchange list suggests one meat exchange. For breakfast, we could add:

　¼ cup cottage cheese

to the 1 cup of milk, 2 Tablespoons raisins, and 1½ cups puffed wheat cereal we chose from the other food groups. What would you choose? Write the answer in your journal.

Dried beans, peas, and lentils are substitutes for meat and are good sources of fiber. A ½-cup serving of these equals one ounce of a medium-fat meat.

Our exchange list for lunch allows two meat exchanges. We could add:

　2 oz. lean roast beef

to the frozen fruit bar and two slices diet bread we chose earlier. What would you choose? Write the answer in your journal.

The dinner exchange list suggests two

meat exchanges. We could add:

2 oz. meatballs

to the 1 cup spaghetti and 1¼ cups straw-berries chosen earlier. What would you choose? Write the answer in your journal.

Remember: One serving of meat generally consists of one ounce of meat, fish, poultry, or cheese. Dried peas and beans are in this group, too.

The vegetable exchanges are also simple. The greatest effort comes from making sure you eat enough of them. Vegetables contain small amounts of carbohydrates and many vitamins and minerals, and are very low in calories. You can consider raw vegetables as a "free" food unless you con-sume more than four cups. Canned vege-table juices are also available. Generally, one serving is ½ cup of cooked vegetables or juice, or 1 cup of raw vegetables.

Examples from the vegetable group include:

asparagus	broccoli
cabbage	carrots
cauliflower	sauerkraut
tomatoes	zucchini

Our exchange list for dinner suggests one vegetable exchange. If we steal the 1 vege-table exchange from lunch, we could add:

½ cup spaghetti sauce (which is 2 vege-table exchanges)

to our earlier choices: 1 cup spaghetti, 2 oz. meatballs, and 1¼ cups strawberries. What would you choose for the vegetable exchanges? Write the answer in your jour-nal.

Remember: The main concern with vegetables is to eat them!

Let's look at fat exchanges. The average North American eats 3 ounces of fat each day. That's like sliding your teeth through eighteen pats of butter at one time! One fat exchange is 1 teaspoon or 5 grams of fat. That's 45 calories per serving.

Nuts, seeds (such as sunflower or sesame), olives, and avocados are high-fat foods and are considered fat exchanges. They are also good sources of vitamins and minerals.

Examples of fat exchanges include:

1 slice bacon (Note: If it's fried crisp, you have crisp fat, not lean bacon!)
1 teaspoon oil, margarine, or butter
8 large olives
1 Tablespoon sunflower seeds
1 teaspoon regular mayonnaise
1 Tablespoon cream cheese
2 Tablespoons sour cream

Fat are also found hidden in food. That's exactly where we will find 2½ of our allowed 3 fat exchanges for the day:

Breakfast
¼ cup cottage cheese = 1 meat exchange and ½ fat exchange

Lunch
2 oz. lean meat = 2 meat exchanges and 1 fat exchange

Dinner
2 oz. meatballs = 2 meat exchanges and 1 fat exchange

We have ¹/2 fat exchange left for the day. We could add:

  4 large olives

to our lunch selections: 2 slices diet bread, 2 oz. lean roast beef, and a frozen fruit bar.

How would you choose to use the day's fat exchanges? Write the answer in your journal.

Remember: Fat calories add up quickly. Select carefully. Use minimal amounts.

The *free* food exchange group won't pass as such in the grocery store checkout! However, these food choices have fewer than 20 calories per serving and can be enjoyed throughout the day with little concern.

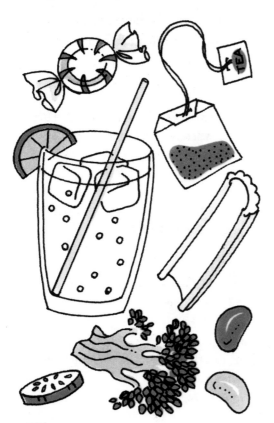

Examples of free foods include:
    sugar-free hard candy
    sugar-free gelatin
    carbonated or mineral water
    calorie-free drink mixes
    coffee, tea
    raw vegetables (less than 4 cups per day)

Remember: Free foods have fewer than 20 calories per serving. Use them to prevent hunger. Snack on these items 30 to 60 minutes before your meal to help you control portions at mealtimes.

Combination foods like casseroles and pizza don't fall into one category. To calculate portions or calories, we need to pull the combination apart and "guesstimate." Food labels of similarly prepared foods will give a breakdown and eliminate some of the guesswork. Ask your dietitian for information on difficult combination foods.

You can do it! Use the lists of the exchange system beginning on page 167 to put together a wide variety of menu choices. It works.

The food guide pyramid

The food guide pyramid is a food planning system developed in 1992 by the U.S. Department of Agriculture (USDA) with support from the U.S. Department of Health and Human Services. The plan divides all food into five groups and assigns another category to fats, oils, and sweets.

Each group in the pyramid has suggested daily servings based on a total calorie intake level. The food pyramid, unlike the exchange system, does not identify the nutrient components (e.g., carbohydrates, fats, proteins) in each group.

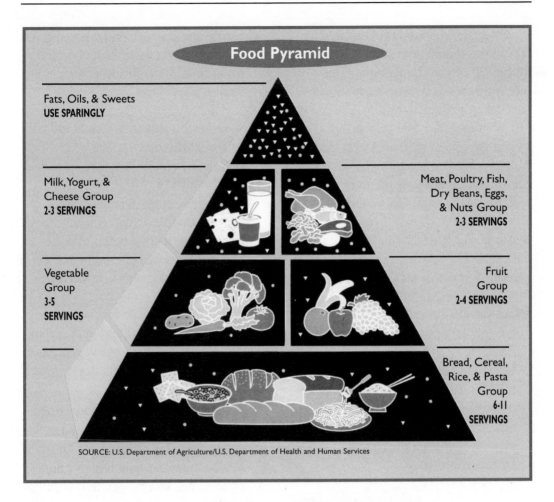

Food Pyramid

Fats, Oils, & Sweets
USE SPARINGLY

**Milk, Yogurt, &
Cheese Group**
2-3 SERVINGS

**Meat, Poultry, Fish,
Dry Beans, Eggs,
& Nuts Group**
2-3 SERVINGS

**Vegetable
Group
3-5
SERVINGS**

**Fruit
Group
2-4 SERVINGS**

**Bread, Cereal,
Rice, & Pasta
Group
6-11
SERVINGS**

SOURCE: U.S. Department of Agriculture/U.S. Department of Health and Human Services

Small circles on the pyramid identify foods with a high fat level. Small triangles on the pyramid identify foods with a high sugar level.

The base of the pyramid shows foods you should eat most frequently. The tip of the pyramid illustrates those that should be eaten the least.

It is appropriate that these guidelines are in a pyramid shape, reminiscent of one of the world's most famous structures. Unfortunately, most people in North America follow a diet that more closely resembles the leaning tower of Pisa.

Let's go through each section of the pyramid in turn.

Fats, oils, and sweets

Fats, oils, and sweets are not considered one of the five groups of healthy choices, and little of your diet should come from this group.

If your goal is to *lose* weight, fat calories should not exceed 25 percent of total intake. This means that a 1,200-calorie diet should have no more than 300 calories from fat (33 fat grams). A 1,500-calorie diet should have no more than 375 calories from fat (42 fat grams). An 1,800-calorie diet should have no more than 450 calories from fat (50 fat grams).

Nutrition and Food Choices

If your goal is to *maintain* your weight, fat calories should not exceed more than 30 percent of your total intake. This means that a 1,200-calorie diet should have no more than 360 calories from fat (40 fat grams). A 1,500-calorie diet should have no more than 450 calories from fat (50 fat grams). An 1,800-calorie diet should have no more than 540 calories from fat (60 fat grams).

Regardless of whether you increase your daily intake of calories, you should not exceed 65 grams of fat a day.

Wise fat choices: the four tips

1. Use low-fat or nonfat spreads.

2. Use low-fat or nonfat salad dressing. If you insist on regular dressing, place it on the side of the plate. Dip your fork in the dressing and then in the salad. You still get the taste but with far fewer calories.

3. Watch out for mayonnaise, which has 100 calories per Tablespoon. Regardless of the brand, mayo has a "standard of identity" law to follow: a certain amount of fat must be present if the product is to be called mayonnaise. Look for products called "lite," "imitation," or "reduced fat." You can find a product with 6 calories per Tablespoon that tastes good. These calorie savings will add up by the time you get to the bottom of the jar. You would consume 2,000 calories in a one-quart jar of nonfat mayo compared to 4,480 calories for a one-quart jar of regular mayonnaise. If you choose the "lite" variety, don't compensate by eating more of it or spreading it more thickly.

4. Use the paper towel test on baked goods. If a food leaves a grease spot on a paper towel, it is obviously high in fat. Pass!

To lose weight, you must closely follow these fat guidelines.

Dairy products

The second tier of the pyramid features foods from animal sources, including dairy products. These dairy products offer vitamins A and D, as well as calcium, but watch out! There are hidden fats in this category.

The food pyramid recommends two to three servings a day, but two servings are ample, especially on a weight-management program of 1,500 calories a day or less.

Wise dairy choices: the four tips

1. Always look for nonfat or low-fat alternatives. Try nonfat milk. One 8-oz. serving of nonfat milk has 85 calories, whereas one serving of whole milk has 150 calories, which means you swallow the equivalent of two pats of butter with each cup.

2. Be choosy with cheese. A 2-oz. serving of American cheese has 212 calories. Substitute low-fat or nonfat alternatives wherever possible. If you do not like the taste of nonfat cheese products, try them when mixing cheese into a recipe and then use regular cheese as a garnish. You have significantly reduced the calories but kept the taste.

3. Select yogurt, both fresh and frozen, with care. Look for low-fat or nonfat yogurt, sweetened with aspartame, to reduce calories.

4. Use low-fat and nonfat sour cream. When cooking, add one teaspoon corn-starch to each cup of sour cream before stirring it into a hot dish, to prevent separation during the cooking process.

Meat, poultry, and fish

The other foods in the second tier of the pyramid are meat, poultry, and fish. All of these are protein-rich foods with other necessary nutrients, including B vitamins, iron, zinc, and phosphorous. (Now you know why you glow in the dark after eating these foods.)

Beans, eggs, and nuts are also included in this section because they are nutritionally similar to fish, meat, and poultry. Nuts and seeds have a high fat content, and egg yolks are high in cholesterol.

The pyramid advises two to three servings a day of these foods. Your total intake for the day, however, should not exceed 7 ounces of meat. These are relatively small servings. For example, in one day you might choose 1/2 medium chicken breast or a palm-sized hamburger as an entree, leaving one to two thin-sliced meats for a sandwich at your light meal.

Wise meat, poultry, and fish choices: the four tips

1. The average 3-pound chicken has 2,600 calories. Skin and fat account for about 70 percent of the total. *Remove the skin before eating.*

2. Trim all fat from red meat prior to cooking.

3. Egg yolks are high in cholesterol, so when cooking, use only one yolk per person. Make up the quantity with egg whites, or simply use egg substitutes.

4. Fish and shellfish are low-fat foods. Fish marinated or fried in oil, however, will be higher in calories. For example, a 6-oz. can of oil-packed tuna has 450 calories while a 6-oz. can of water-packed tuna has 220 calories.

Vegetables

In the third layer of the pyramid you will find fruit and vegetables. The recommendation is three to five servings per day of vegetables. Vegetables contain many important nutrients, including vitamin A, beta carotene, vitamins C and K, folacin, iron, and magnesium. These nutrients are essential for health. Although it is possible to get some of these nutrients in multi-vitamin tablets, there is no substitute for eating the vegetables themselves. For example, beta carotene is just one of over 400 carotenoids found in carrots. Taking beta carotene in pill form, therefore, is not the same as eating a carrot.

In terms of nutrition, there is no difference between fresh and frozen vegetables.

The calorie content of vegetables is negligible, and there is no need to worry about the volume of vegetables you eat. The only way that lettuce would be damaging is if a ton of it fell on top of you.

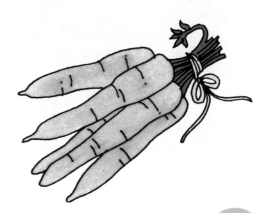

Wise vegetable choices: the four tips

1. Use fresh vegetables as snacks. Carry them with you to munch while on the go. Broccoli, cauliflower, and carrots make good snacks and should be part of your salads, too.

2. Make sure that any toppings you use are low-fat or nonfat. Stay away from added butter, cheese, and cream sauces. Try salsa as a topping for baked potatoes.

3. Use flavored vinegars (have you tried raspberry vinegar?) for healthy and tasty salad dressings.

4. Use vegetable, tomato, and carrot juices as refreshing drinks.

Fruits

As with vegetables, fruits contain many essential nutrients and are a good source of fiber. The recommendation is two to four servings a day. The size of the fruit is important. One medium banana counts as two servings, as does one large apple. If you are hungry, fruit makes a great snack.

Wise fruit choices: the four tips

1. Although fruit juices are a healthy choice, they do contain significant calories. Each $1/4$ to $1/2$ cup (depending on the fruit) provides the same number of calories as the whole fruit. One solution is to take a small amount of fruit juice and add it to sparkling water for a refreshing drink.

2. Dried fruits make a healthy snack. Be careful, however. The water was "dried," not the calories! Check labels for serving size and calories.

3. If you want a pureed fruit snack that is low in calories, try a jar of baby food.

4. Frozen fruit makes a refreshing snack, especially in summer. Try frozen grapes or slices of frozen banana or pineapple.

Bread, cereal, pasta, and rice

As these foods form the foundation of the pyramid, they should form the basis of your meal plan. These foods are rich in minerals, vitamins, and fiber. They should make up the bulk of caloric intake.

The food pyramid recommendation is six to eleven servings a day, depending on your overall intake. If you are on a 1,200-calorie-a-day diet, the recommendation is five servings. For a 1,500-calorie-a-day plan, eight servings are recommended.

Wise bread, cereal, pasta, and rice choices: the four tips

1. Watch out! Portion sizes are conservative. One serving equals:

    1 slice of bread
    $1/2$ hot dog or hamburger bun
    $1/2$ cup potato or rice or pasta
    4 to 6 small cracker squares

2. Read the label on cereal boxes for serving size and calorie counts. Some cereals contain coconut or nuts that can make the calorie count jump.

3. Avoid cheese, cream, and other high-fat sauces on pasta and rice.

4. Measure out cereal. It's easy to pile up too much in the bowl.

A typical day's menu with a 1,200-calorie limit puts you at the low end of the number of portions suggested by the pyramid. A typical day's menu could be:

Breakfast:
   3/4 cup bran flakes
   1 cup nonfat milk
   1 small banana

Lunch:
   Sandwich:
      2 slices whole-wheat bread
      2 oz. fat-free sandwich meat
      1 tsp. fat-free mayonnaise
   Raw veggies: carrot "pennies"
      1/2 sliced green pepper
      Raw cauliflower

Dinner:
   1 cup pasta mixed with
      1 cup steamed broccoli flowerettes
   1/2 grilled chicken breast
   1/2 cup low-fat frozen yogurt

Snacks:
   1 small apple
   2 medium breadsticks

EXERCISE:
In your journal, write
two days' menus using
the serving sizes recommended
for each food group in the pyramid.
Use the low end of the range
listed in each area.

For the purposes of weight management, we recommend:

   6 to 8 servings from the bread, cereal, rice, and pasta group
   2 to 3 servings from the fruit group
   3 to 5 servings from the vegetable group
   2 servings from the dairy group
   6 to 7 ounces from the meat, poultry, and fish group
   And. . . unlimited servings from the support group (your TOPS chapter).

You can do it! The choice is yours!

The "plate method"
This is a simple visual method of portion control.

Mark off one half of your dinner plate. This is the space for vegetables. Divide the other half in two. One half of this half of the plate is for potato, rice, or pasta and the other half is for meat, poultry, or fish. It's a quick and easy diet plan!

Vitamins and minerals
Although the clerk at your local health food store claims it's essential to load up on megadoses of vitamins and other "botanicals" to lose weight, stay young, and improve your sex life, the fact is that a balanced diet is sufficient for optimal health. Promoters of dietary supplements often mislead consumers. There is no need to invest your week's wages in a special multivitamin formula derived especially from the floor of the Brazilian rainforest when fruit from your local supermarket will do just as well, if not better.

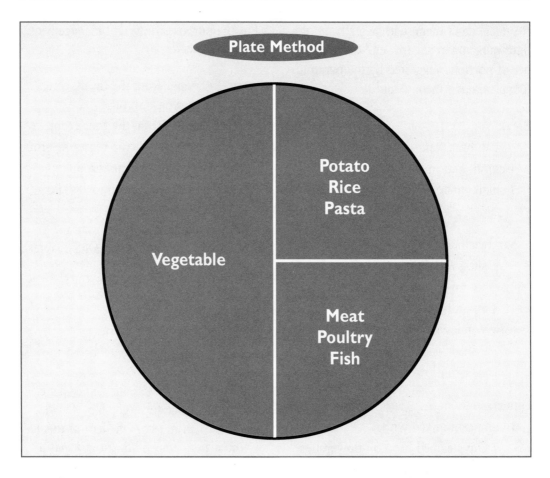

Plate Method

Vegetable

Potato
Rice
Pasta

Meat
Poultry
Fish

Not only is there no need to take excess vitamins and minerals (unless specifically advised by your physician), but mega-dosing can create problems. For example, excessive amounts of vitamin D may cause calcification of soft tissue. Excessive vitamin C may mask symptoms of disease and contribute to kidney stone development.

How do I know I am getting all the vitamins I need?

Let's take a closer look at vitamins and where you find them. See the tables on pages 54 and 55. Although seeking out these nutrients may seem like one more onerous responsibility, if you are eating a sensible, healthy diet as outlined in this guide, you will be meeting your requirements.

There are two categories of vitamins:
• Fat-soluble vitamins
  (dissolve in fat)
• Water-soluble vitamins
  (dissolve in water)

Some substances, such as para-amino benzoic acid, citrus bioflavonoid complex, hesperidin, and pangamic acid, have been termed "vitamins" by self-proclaimed experts. They are of no known importance in human nutrition. Their absence from the diet does not cause disease.

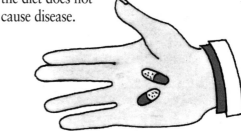

Will I get all the minerals I need on my weight-control program?

Most definitely, yes! By eating a variety of foods, in moderation, you will achieve an adequate intake.

Your most important strategy is to avoid all excesses or deficiencies of vitamins, minerals, or any other food compound that becomes hyped.

Minerals

Let's look at some of the minerals and note how easy it would be to routinely include them in your diet. See the table on pages 56 and 57.

A balanced diet provides most necessary vitamins and minerals. Supplementation is rarely necessary and should never be undertaken without medical advice.

What are phytochemicals?

Phytochemicals are chemicals from plants. All foods, even spices, have thousands of phytochemicals, many of which have yet to be identified. Some phytochemicals may have a role in the prevention of disease, but at this point there is no recommendation for supplementing individual phytochemicals. These are not magic potions, regardless of what the clerk in your health food store may tell you.

Beta carotene was one of the first antioxidants to hit the market. It gives fruits and vegetables their yellow/orange color and may have a role in preventing heart and lung disease. Some studies, however, do not demonstrate any disease risk reduction with these supplements. Where positive results have been demonstrated, it is only the consumption of food containing beta carotene, not beta carotene supplements, that resulted in substantial reduction in risk of cancer and heart disease. Beta carotene can be found in carrots, and so can 400 other carotenoids.

PRACTICAL TIP:
Eat at least five carrots a week.

Isoflavones are the plant equivalent of the female hormone lost at menopause. Soy foods are a good source. This phytochemical has been shown to provide relief from troublesome symptoms of menopause and can also reduce serum cholesterol levels. Two to three servings of soy foods per day can decrease cholesterol levels, and just one serving can reduce the risk of cancer.

PRACTICAL TIPS:
Use low-fat soy milk in place of regular milk in cooking or on cereal.
Use soy flour when baking.
Use textured vegetable protein in place of ground beef.

Fat-Soluble Vitamins

Vitamin/Role	Recommended amount	Sources
VITAMIN A Involved in the formation and maintenance of skin and mucous membranes. Increases resistance to infections and allows us to see at night by adjusting to changes in light.	5,000 IU (international units)	There are two forms of vitamin A, each with its own food sources: RETINOL: liver, butter, whole milk, cheese, and egg yolk PRO-VITAMIN A: carrots, leafy green vegetables, sweet potatoes, pumpkin, winter squash, mango, and papaya
VITAMIN D Builds bones and teeth, and regulates calcium.	400 IU	Vitamin-D-fortified milk and other dairy products, fish oils, egg yolk, sunshine (four hours in two weeks will meet the requirement)
VITAMIN E An antioxidant which prevents some body cells from harming other tissues of the body.	12 to 15 IU	Vegetable oil, margarine, nuts, leafy green vegetables, wheat germ, whole-grain products, liver, and egg yolk
VITAMIN K Allows blood to clot.	60 to 80 micrograms a day	Broccoli, sweet and hot peppers, collards, Brussels sprouts, strawberries, oranges, kale, grapefruit, potatoes, tomatoes, spinach, and tangerines

Water-Soluble Vitamins

Vitamin/Role	Recommended amount	Sources
VITAMIN B$_1$ (THIAMINE) Aids in normal body structure and function. Helps body break down fruit, starch, and milk.	1.5 mg (milligrams)	Whole grains, fortified grain products, pork, liver, legumes, and nuts
VITAMIN B$_2$ (RIBOFLAVIN) Aids in cell function, especially with the body's use of fat. Promotes good vision & healthy skin.	Men: 1.4 to 1.7 mg per day Women: 1.2 to 1.3 mg per day	Milk, yogurt, cottage cheese, liver, meat, and fortified grain products

Vitamin/Role	Recommended amount	Sources
NIACIN Aids in body's use of fat & carbohydrate. Promotes healthy skin, nerves, & digestive system.	Men: 15 to 19 mg per day Women: 13 to 15 mg per day	Meat, poultry, fish, peanuts, fortified grain products, tuna, and asparagus
Note: Larger amounts of niacin are sometimes used to control blood cholesterol. These high levels can contribute to some side effects. Niacin taken for this purpose should be monitored by a physician.		
FOLACIN Promotes red blood cell formation.	180 to 200 mg per day	Legumes, leafy green vegetables, meats, sprouts, and orange juice
VITAMIN B6 (PYRIDOXINE) Helps the body use protein. Assists in red blood cell formation.	Men: 2 mg per day Women: 1.6 mg per day	Beans, bananas, breads, eggs, fish, legumes, meat, and nuts
Note: B6 is often promoted as a "necessary supplement" in some markets. Intake which exceeds the recommendation may result in irreversible nerve damage.		
VITAMIN B12 Assists in formation of red blood cells and maintenance of nerve tissue.	2 micrograms per day	Meat, poultry, fish, shellfish, milk, milk products, and organ meats
BIOTIN Aids in the metabolism of fat and carbohydrate.	30 to 100 micrograms per day	Organ meats, milk, egg yolks, most fresh vegetables, yeast, peanuts, and cheese
PANTOTHENIC ACID Involved in energy metabolism.	4 to 7 mg per day	Meat, organ meats, whole grains, legumes, egg yolks, and mushrooms
VITAMIN C Develops collagen fibers which strengthen tissues, helps bones and blood vessels, promotes wound healing, has an antioxidant role of protecting body from the harmful effects of "free radicals."	60 mg per day Smokers should take 100 mg per day. (They should also quit smoking immediately.)	Green peppers, broccoli, collards, Brussels sprouts, oranges, strawberries, kale, grapefruit, potatoes, mango, spinach, tomatoes, and tangerines

Lycopene, which is found in tomatoes, has been related to decreased risk for prostate and mouth cancer. Regular tomato eaters cut in half their risk for cancer of the digestive tract. Studies suggest consuming ten tomatoes a week to get these benefits.

PRACTICAL TIPS:
Use tomato paste in recipes
(small can = five tomatoes).
Use tomato sauce on vegetables and pasta (small can = two tomatoes).
Keep a bowl of cherry tomatoes handy for snacks.

Minerals

Mineral/Role	Recommended amount	Sources
SODIUM Maintains water balance. Essential for nerve and muscle functions.	500 mg per day (That's only $1/4$ teaspoon of salt; and remember that there are also many natural sources.)	Table salt, preservatives in frozen meals and packaged "instant" products, celery, and softened water
POTASSIUM Maintains water balance. Essential for nerve and muscle function.	2,000 mg per day	Prevalent in most foods, especially fruit and vegetables
Note: Deficiencies can occur from illnesses that cause vomiting or diarrhea, or from use of diuretics. Potassium supplements should not be taken without medical advice.		
CHLORIDE Forms hydrochloric acid in the stomach to aid digestion.	200 mg per day	Table salt
Note: The average North American consumes 700 times the daily recommended intake of chloride through use of table salt.		
PHOSPHOROUS Provides bone growth, strength, and maintenance.	800 mg per day	Dairy foods, bakery products, and meat
Note: The average North American consumes $1 1/2$ times the daily recommended intake of phosphorous–more if soda is a daily beverage.		

Mineral/Role	Recommended amount	Sources
CALCIUM Bone growth and development	1,000 to 1,500 mg per day	Dairy products & soybean products

Note: If caloric restrictions prevent you from drinking three or more glasses of milk a day, ask your physician about a calcium supplement. Guidance in choosing a supplement is necessary because some contain significant amounts of lead, which can be poisonous.

Note: Estrogen plays an important role in the absorption of calcium, so postmenopausal women are at high risk for deficiency.

Mineral/Role	Recommended amount	Sources
MAGNESIUM Bone growth and development	Men: 350 mg per day Women: 280 mg per day	Drinking water (except softened water from which calcium and magnesium are removed), whole grains, broccoli, squash, beans, nuts, seeds, and dairy products

Note: If you are postmenopausal and taking calcium supplements, this may limit the amount of magnesium absorbed in your system. Discuss a blood measurement with your physician.

Mineral/Role	Recommended amount	Sources
IRON Development of red blood cells and muscles	Men: 10 mg per day Women: 15 mg per day	Red meat, enriched grains and cereals, and oysters

Note: Iron is difficult for the body to absorb. Eating it with a food rich in vitamin C (e.g., by including tomatoes in your salad) will increase absorption.

Mineral/Role	Recommended amount	Sources
ZINC Controls growth, sexual maturation, wound healing, maintenance of skin, hair, nails, and mucous membranes of the mouth, throat, stomach, and intestines.	Men: 15 mg per day Women: 12 mg per day	Lean meat, organ meat, seafood, dairy products, and whole grains
SELENIUM Protects the heart against oxidation by "free radicals."	55 to 70 micrograms	Fish, meat, eggs, shellfish, and whole grains
CHROMIUM Aids glucose uptake.	2 to 5 mg per day	Whole grains and meats, and fresh fruits

Elegiac acid and veritol are found in nuts. Nuts also contain the amino acid arginine, vitamin E, and folic acid. If you are nuts about nuts (that is, if you consume nuts at least five times a week), you probably reduce your risk of coronary artery disease by 50 percent, but you might also ruin your weight-control program because nuts are a concentrated source of calories and monounsaturated fat.

PRACTICAL TIP:
Try one ounce of nuts a day, and eat them instead of another food with high fat content.

Organosulfides, which can be found in onions, provide protection against stomach and colon cancer. Garlic, also included in this group, reduces cholesterol, blood pressure, and blood clots. A little garlic a day may keep more than your friends away.

PRACTICAL TIP:
Eat half an onion and one clove of garlic daily.

Flavonoids, of which tea is the main source, can decrease heart disease and cancer.

PRACTICAL TIP:
Have a cup of green or black tea in the morning and in the afternoon.

Anthocyanins, which is Greek for "blue flower," are antioxidants that fight heart disease and cancer. They can be found in purple cabbages and grapes.

PRACTICAL TIPS:
Add purple cabbage to salads.
Have frozen grapes as snacks.

As you can see, a diet that is high in fruit, vegetables, and starches, as the exchange system recommends, includes all the vitamins, minerals, and phytochemicals currently known to be beneficial.

Strategies for shopping

Don't go grocery shopping when you are hungry. If there is ever an example of the relationship between physical state and behavior, this is it. When you shop hungry, you end up buying foods you don't need.

Always make a list. If you have a list, you are far less likely to "wing it" and end up with foods you had not planned on.

Go to a store that you know, if at all possible. That way you need not wander down every aisle to find what you want. The longer you stay in a grocery store, the more likely you are to deviate from your list. Arrange your list in the order you shop. Less roaming will reduce temptation.

It may be easier to go to the store more often to get just a few items each time. Less time is spent in the store per visit, so there is less opportunity for losing focus.

Include a variety of foods on your shopping list. More than 2,000 foods are available in a typical supermarket, yet most people tend to repeat the same purchases week after week, limiting themselves to about 200 items. Don't get into a boring rut! Vary your shopping with seasonal foods. Make one new purchase each time you shop.

Don't be too quick to substitute an item on your list. If you cannot find a particular food, ask employees for help.

Foods in the dietetic section can be expensive and unnecessary.

Use any device to keep you mindful of your weight management efforts. Use your motivational imagery or tokens. Wear tight clothing. Make an audiotape of your reasons for losing weight, and listen to it as you go around the store.

Strategies for food preparation

Don't snack while you are preparing food. Put away the ingredients after use so they are not sitting on the counter waiting to be eaten.

If necessary, eat a small snack (fruit, vegetables, or even cereal) before preparing a meal so you are not hungry while cooking.

Avoid drinking alcohol while cooking. As you have already learned, alcohol stimulates appetite, and this will create a tempting situation.

Tasting is meant to be just that—tasting, not eating half a portion. Tea tasters take a small sip and then spit it out, and you could

do the same. (Be sure that your dinner guests are not watching when you do this!)

Make just enough for the number of people you will be serving. There's no need to make extra just in case three people suddenly drop by.

If you're cooking for more than one meal, freeze the rest. Ideally, freeze the rest in individual portion sizes. Also, do this before you sit down to eat, if at all possible. If you wander back into the kitchen just after eating and there is food sitting out, it will tempt you.

Make sure you serve plenty of fruits, vegetables, and bread (watch the butter!) to fill the gap just in case three people do drop in unexpectedly.

Cooking tips that make a difference

- Steam, bake, poach, or grill instead of frying.

- Stir-fry, using small amounts of oil.

- Prepare all meat low-fat. Trim away visible fat. Lay the trimmed fat on the grill away from the meat—the fat drippings and the smoke that rises will enhance the meat flavor.

- In casseroles, use less meat. In its place, use extra vegetables and extra pasta or rice.

- Marinate meat, fish, or poultry in a fat-free Italian dressing for added flavor.

- Seal in the natural juices of some food by wrapping in foil or edible pouches (e.g., cabbage leaves) before steaming, baking, or poaching.

- Maintain maximum flavor by cooking to the tender-crisp stage. Broccoli can't swim.

- Remove some of the salt or fat from canned goods. Drain the oil or brine, add water to the can, drain and rinse again.

- Toast seeds, nuts, or whole spices to enhance flavor. Bake on a cookie sheet or pie tin at 400°F until browned.

- Flavored vinegars add a tangy flavor to vegetables and fish. Balsamic vinegar is great. Add at the last minute.

- Dry mustard mixed with water adds spice and "bite."

- Dried mushrooms, tomatoes, and chilies are full of flavor. Soften them in a small amount of water, which you can then use to add extra flavor with few extra calories.

- Add a drop of lemon juice to the cooking water for rice and pasta. Forget the salt.

- Keep a pack of gum in the cupboard closest to your cooking area. Chew gum while cooking to avoid excessive food tasting.

- Make soups, stews, and gravies ahead of time so they can be chilled and excess fat removed.

- When possible, use brown rice. It has more flavor than white rice.

- Fresh herbs and whole spices have more flavor than dried ones. Grate fresh ginger, and use a processor for horseradish. Add fresh herbs just before serving.

- Try fresh citrus "zest." Remove the peel of an orange, grapefruit, or lemon, cut into strips, and use on poultry or fish.

Portions
How do they Measure Up?

A 4-ounce portion of raw meat is about the size of your palm or the size of a deck of cards.

A small apple or orange is about the size of a tennis ball.

A thumbnail is roughly equivalent to 1 teaspoon. A thumb is about an ounce.

An ounce of cheese is one 1" cube.

- Try one of the salt-free spice blends.

- Make your own version of macaroni and cheese with fat-free shredded cheese and low-fat milk. Sprinkle regular cheese on top. No one will know!

Strategies for portion control

One of the biggest problems on a weight-management program is managing portion sizes. This is especially true when eating out, because restaurant portions can be large. Ways of managing portion size when you are eating out include:

- Specifying portion size
- Splitting entrees
- Ordering a child-sized or senior portion
- Constructing a meal out of appetizers

Know what your portions are and what they look like.

Keys to portion control

- Obtain measuring cups and spoons and a food scale. They are necessary for accurate measurement.

- Serve your usual portion of food. Now measure it. Was it more or less than expected? Will your usual portion fit into your meal plan?

- Measure margarine, milk for cereal, gravy, sauces, and salad dressings before you serve them.

- If measuring devices are not available, the hand method is a good alternative. A palm (not including fingers) is equivalent to 4 ounces of raw meat. A fist equals about 1 cup of liquid, a small potato, or 1 cup of pasta or rice. A thumbnail is roughly equivalent to 1 teaspoon, and a thumb is about an ounce.

- Portions of meat, fish, or poultry can be weighed before or after cooking. Four ounces of raw meat will become 3 ounces when cooked.

- Look at the serving size on food labels. Then measure the amount that fits into your plan. With practice, you will be able to "eyeball" the right amount.

- Use the same size mug, glass, or bowl each day. Measure so you'll know how far to fill your mug to meet, and not exceed, your requirements.

Strategies for snacking

On some occasions, snacking is an appropriate method of hunger control.

Snacking should always be planned. Scheduling a mid-morning or afternoon snack to head off hunger until mealtime is a useful strategy. Such snacks, as part of a program of small, frequent meals, keep your blood glucose levels on an even keel.

Never let yourself get really hungry. Healthy snacks will prevent you from getting into this situation. Have healthy snacks like fruit, cereal, or vegetables easily available for times when a healthy lunch or meal is not possible.

Snacks should consist mainly of complex carbohydrates. They should never exceed 200 calories.

Find a kitchen shelf to house low-fat, low-calorie snack items.

Keep a corner of the fridge ready with items to grab.

Snacks can be destructive to your weight-management program when they are:
- Unplanned
- High in calories
- High in sugar (This is likely to prime further, uncontrolled consumption.)

Good Snack Suggestions
Cup-of-soup

Sardines or shrimp
   in spring water

Melba toast

Rice cakes

Mini bagels

Fruit Roll-Ups

Applesauce
   (in individual containers)

Fig bars

Pretzels

Popcorn

Fat-free yogurt

Frozen fruit bars

Sorbet

Sugar-free frozen treats

Raw vegetables

Remember to keep those snacks under 200 calories.

Strategies for restaurants
Many people eat more than half their meals away from home. If you frequently eat out, it is important to be able to manage your program in a restaurant.

Some things you can do even before you get to the restaurant are:

- Choose a restaurant where you know you can get a healthy meal. If you are unsure or are in unfamiliar territory, call ahead to determine whether the restaurant can meet your needs.

- Avoid buffet style, all-you-can-eat restaurants.

- Go with people who are supportive and won't sabotage your plan, willingly or otherwise ("friendly enemies").

- Determine ahead of time what you are going to order.

- Don't go hungry. Have a healthy snack a couple of hours beforehand.

When you get to the restaurant:

- As soon as you sit down, order a salad and a glass of water or soda. Waiting for your meal to arrive is difficult, so it's important to have something to fill this time.

- Order first, so you are not influenced by the rest of your party.

- If you already know what you are having, don't even look at the menu.

- Be assertive. Control portion size by splitting an entree, ordering appetizers, ordering half-portions or specifying a particular amount (e.g., "just four ounces, please!")

- Remove the bread from the table, or at least remove it from your end of the table.

- Have sauces and dressings served on the side.

- Dip your fork into the sauce or dressing and then into the food, not the other way around. You get the taste of the dressing but eat far less of it.

- Watch the alcohol. Remember, willpower dissolves in alcohol. If you're having wine, order it by the glass.

Calorie Content of Some Alcoholic Beverages

Beverage	Calories
12 oz. lite beer	100
12 oz. regular beer	150
12 oz. nonalcoholic beer	60
4 oz. dry white wine	85
4 oz. sweet wine	105
12 oz. wine cooler	215
1 1/2 oz. gin, rum, vodka, whiskey, or brandy	100
1 1/2 oz. liqueur	160
4 oz. daiquiri	220
5 oz. Bloody Mary	115

Strategies for fast food restaurants

Fast food restaurants create special problems for the weight-conscious person. Generally, the food is high in fat and not a good choice. On the other hand, fast food restaurants are popular because they are convenient.

DID YOU KNOW?

The average time taken to consume a double-size burger, french fries, and a milkshake is just $4\frac{1}{2}$ minutes. During this short period, consumption would total about 1,500 calories.

Salads are always a healthy choice, but watch out for the salad dressing, the bacon bits, and the croutons. Check the portion size of the salad dressing—it often contains more calories than the salad itself.

Roasted or broiled meat and chicken sandwiches can be a good choice. Substitute mustard for mayonnaise.

Baked potatoes are good. Try to have them plain, or top them with a very small amount of margarine or sour cream.

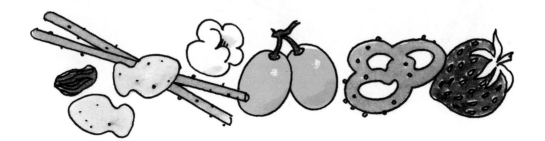

A regular plain hamburger is acceptable. Again, watch out for the mayo. A plain hamburger is about your allowance of red meat for the day. Double and triple burgers exceed the recommendations for red meat allowances in a single stroke.

If you're ordering pizza, have it plain or loaded with vegetables instead of pepperoni.

PRACTICAL TIP:
Avoiding fried foods cuts your calorie consumption by 75 percent. A typical double cheeseburger, fries, and shake provide 1,520 calories. A broiled chicken sandwich, salad with fat-free dressing, and diet soda provide fewer than 400 calories.

Strategies for dinner parties

Being a guest can present problems, especially if you are not well acquainted with your host or hostess. Some strategies can help.

If you know the host well, offer to bring a dish of your own—ostensibly for everyone else, but also for you. With this tactic, many vegetarians quite comfortably survive dining out.

If you do not know your hostess well:

• Make the best choices you can.

• Limit yourself to small portions.

• Don't be self-conscious. Most of the others there are in the same situation. It is unlikely that anybody is scrutinizing what and how much you eat.

• Always be polite. You can say no graciously.

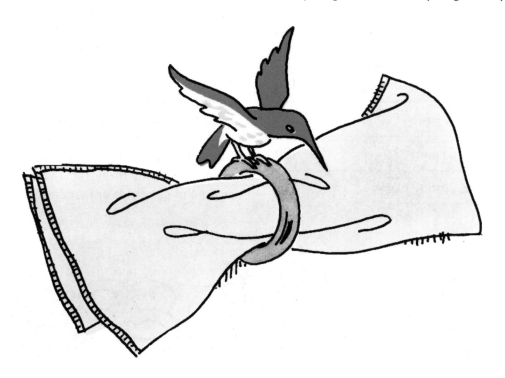

- If absolutely necessary, take what is offered and push it around your plate, slip it to the dog, drop it in the vase, or throw it out the window.

Don't be militant. Don't be judgmental about the food. Don't be a nutritional know-it-all. Even if the food is high in fat and nutritionally poor, you do not have to give a wellness commentary.

If you are declining dessert (or anything else), just say "no, thank you." Don't create elaborate excuses for why you cannot eat the food.

Try not to keep food in front of you. Once you have finished eating, move away from the table and the food, if at all possible.

Strategies for parties and other special events

You can have a good time at parties and other special events. You will feel better if you make better choices. Ways of doing this include:

- Arrive late and leave early to minimize your exposure.

- Stay away from the food table. Hovering around the food will make it too difficult to resist.

- Don't go hungry. Have a meal or at least a snack before you go.

- Focus on the social aspects of the occasion.

- Keep a drink (preferably water or diet soda) in your hand. If you choose to drink alcohol, consider spritzers; also, alternate alcoholic drinks with non-alcoholic ones. Non-alcoholic wines and beers are also good choices.

Strategies for traveling

Traveling presents particular problems because you are often thrown off your normal schedule, you're in unfamiliar places, and your normal exercise routine may be disrupted.

Remember, a golden rule of managing high-risk situations is *never go hungry.* For that reason, it is important to have healthy snacks available at all times.

If you are traveling by car, especially on a long trip:

- Take along a cooler in which you can keep water, diet sodas, fruit, low-fat yogurt, and other healthy snacks. Pretzels make a good travel snack, as does dry cereal.

- Plan your stops. If you are going to stop at a fast food restaurant, plan ahead of time what you will order.

- Stop every couple of hours to fight off fatigue and prevent stiffness.

- Watch out for gas station food. Ninety-five percent of it is high-fat!

- Make sandwiches to take with you.

If you are traveling on a plane:

- Take snacks with you. You never know when, where, and for how long you may be delayed.

- Watch out for nuts served as in-flight snacks.

- If there is an in-flight meal, order a special meal up to twenty-four hours before departure. Various good alternatives include the fruit plate and the diabetic meals. The vegetarian meal can be high in fat. Once you have ordered a special meal, don't change your seat assignment or you may go hungry!

When in an unfamiliar place:

• Find out in advance as much as possible about local restaurants.

• Ask the locals about places that serve healthy food (assuming the locals know what healthy food is!)

• Even on vacation, there's no reason to abandon your usual sensible habits.

— Specify portion sizes.

— Keep sauces and dressings on the side.

— Minimize the fat; ask for grilled foods.

— Choose mainly chicken and fish.

— Watch out for desserts.

— Request bottled mineral water in places that don't have diet sodas.

• Cruises offer a wonderful selection of fruits and vegetables as well as vegetarian cuisine.

• Many hotels offer a buffet breakfast with fruit, cereal, and a selection of breads.

Nutrition quiz

1) How many calories are there in a gram of unsaturated fat?
2) How do saturated fats differ from unsaturated ones?
3) What is the daily calorie allowance on the typical food label?
4) What is the recommended daily intake of vitamin E?
5) How many calories are there in a Tablespoon of mayonnaise?

Answers:
1) 9 calories
2) Saturated fats are more harmful to health.
3) 2,000
4) 12-15 IU
5) 100

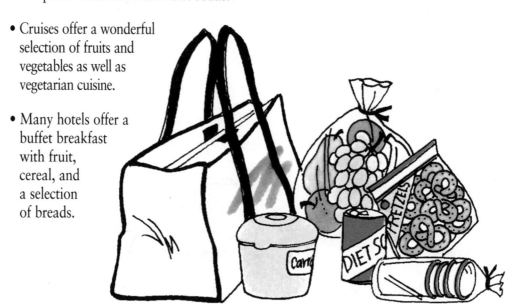

EXERCISE AND PHYSICAL FITNESS

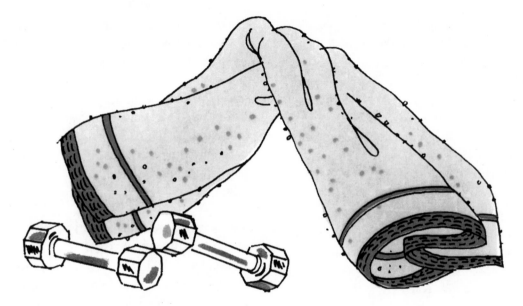

A good exercise routine is an essential part of any weight-control program. Not only does it account for increased caloric expenditure but it also has significant psychological and physical benefits.

In this section you will learn:

- About the importance of exercise and physical fitness
- Why you must exercise to manage your weight
- What sorts of exercise to do
- How to design your own exercise program
- Good exercise practices and answers to common questions
- How to assess cardiovascular fitness, flexibility, and strength

The importance of exercise and physical fitness

Physical fitness is defined as the body's ability to adapt to the demands and stresses of physical effort. The President's Council on Physical Fitness defines fitness as the ability to carry out daily tasks without undue fatigue and to have ample energy to enjoy leisure pursuits and avoid or quickly recover from unexpected injuries.

The more we ask of our bodies, the stronger and more fit they become. The less we ask of them, the less they can do. In a world that depends more and more on labor-saving technology, we have become far less active. This inactivity contributes to obesity. To develop and maintain physical fitness, we have to make a special effort to include it in daily life.

The benefits of exercise

We have seen that there are no magic solutions; there is a price to pay for using medications. But suppose there was a drug that could give you all of these benefits:

- Reduced disease risk
- Positive mood
- Improved cardiovascular performance
- Increased stamina
- Increased endurance
- Increased energy
- Increased metabolism
- Burning of calories
- Reduced health risks
- Preservation of muscle mass
- Preservation of bone mass
- Toning of muscle
- Stress reduction
- Faster recovery time from illness and injury

If a company claimed its drug could do all this, either you would not believe it or you would head straight to the drugstore, clutching your prescriptions to your chest.

The truth is that there is no drug that can do this, but exercise can. Of course it is easier to simply pop a pill than to take a 30-minute walk, but then again, that's part of the power of the exercise: *Its benefits come from your own effort.*

There is no question that if you want to do just one thing to enhance your quality of life, exercise is it (unless you're a smoker, in which case your number one priority should be quitting smoking). The beauty of exercise is that not only is it essential to a good weight-management program but it is also essential to overall physical and mental health.

Why you must exercise to manage your weight

As you have already learned, weight loss only occurs when your caloric expenditure exceeds your caloric intake. If you just focus on reducing your caloric intake, unfortunately your caloric expenditure decreases too. How does this happen?

If a person is inactive, muscle mass declines. This is important because muscle mass increases the body's rate of metabolism. Building muscle mass, or at the very least preserving it, is critical in maintaining body metabolism and thus caloric expenditure. Of course, exercise burns calories in its own right. During exercise, metabolic rate is increased, and *this increase is sustained for several hours after the workout.*

68

Several studies have clearly demonstrated that following a sensible diet and exercise program is the best way of losing fat and keeping it off.

Is there a difference between fat and weight?

While you are concerned with your overall weight, what you are really trying to manage is your fat. If you do not exercise, your low-calorie diet will produce the loss of some fat *and some muscle*. If you combine a sensible diet with an exercise program, you will lose more fat and less muscle.

Let's look at an example. Suppose your friend goes on a restrictive low-calorie diet, does not exercise, and loses 12 pounds—8 pounds of fat and 4 pounds of muscle.

You, being a well-informed person, follow a program of sensible diet and exercise. You lose 10 pounds of fat but *gain* 1 pound of muscle—a total of 9 pounds lost. Who is better off?

Your friend might feel temporarily superior, but she is asking for trouble in the future. She has reduced her metabolism and lost muscle mass. Her chances of maintaining a very-low-calorie diet are poor. Sooner rather than later, she is likely to increase calorie consumption and regain her weight. The regained weight will be fat, so overall through this diet cycle she has exchanged 4 pounds of muscle for 4 pounds of fat.

You, on the other hand, have a much more manageable program. The exercise will make you feel better and will increase your metabolism and burn calories. Even if you deviate a little from your nutrition program from time to time, the exercise will protect against weight regain.

What sort of exercise should I do?

There are three types of exercise: aerobic, resistance, and flexibility. All of them are important for a well-rounded weight-management program. Please check with your doctor before beginning any exercise routine.

Aerobic exercise

Aerobic activity is designed to benefit the cardiorespiratory system—the heart and lungs. Only aerobic activities will help increase cardiovascular endurance, which is the ability of heart and lungs to take in and transport oxygen to the muscles for activities performed over a long period of time. In fact, the word aerobic means "with air."

Aerobic activities get the heart rate into a certain range, about 65 to 75 percent of its peak capacity. There is an easy way to calculate this "target heart rate" that constitutes the aerobic range. To calculate your target heart rate, begin by determining your maximum heart rate. Do this by subtracting your age from 220. Thus, for someone 40 years old, the maximum heart rate is $220 - 40 = 180$.

Your aerobic range is 60 to 75 percent of the maximum heart rate. To continue our example, 60 percent of 180 = 108 beats per minute; and 75 percent of 180 = 135 beats per minute. Therefore, this person's target heart rate range is 108 to 135 beats per minute.

Some medications keep heart rate low and make it necessary to revise the target heart rate range. For example, some of the medications used to treat high blood pressure or heart disease can reduce target heart rate. Consult with your physician about your particular target heart rate if you are taking medication for these conditions.

How do I know that I have reached my target heart range?

A 10-second sampling of your pulse gives an adequate measure of overall heart rate. In 10 seconds, you will count one-sixth of your per-minute heart rate. If your target heart rate range is 108 to 135 beats per minute, a 10-second pulse of 18 to 22 beats per minute would confirm that you are indeed in your range.

I want to be an exerciser, not a paramedic. Do I really have to keep taking my pulse?

No. Actually, taking your pulse can be disruptive and can interfere with your enjoyment of the exercise. If you wish to check it periodically as a matter of interest, that's fine, but you don't have to stop frequently to monitor your heart rate. If you like constant feedback, several manufacturers make heart rate monitors that will give you a continuous pulse reading.

The perceived exertion scale is another way to check your exercise level, and it provides a better overall guide than heart rate.

The perceived exertion scale

As your exercise progresses, you will become familiar with the amount of effort required to raise your heart rate to target levels. In other words, you will know how you feel when you have exercised intensely enough. At this point, you can use the perceived exertion scale—an estimate of how hard you are working during exercise —to reach and maintain your intensity in future workouts. Exercise hard enough to reach the same level of exertion.

The Perceived Exertion Scale

Very easy
No change in pulse from resting level

Easy/Somewhat easy
Little change or slight increase in pulse and breathing

Moderate
Modest increase in pulse and breathing

Somewhat difficult/Difficult
Heavy breathing and sweating

Very difficult
Sustained heavy breathing and sweating

You should aim to keep yourself in the "moderate" range and never get beyond "somewhat difficult."

PRACTICAL TIP:
A simple measure of exertion is that if you cannot hold a conversation during your workout, you are exercising too hard.

Aerobic Aqua Exercises

BOBBING
Standing in shallow water, inhale and duck under water to a squat position. Push off the bottom of the pool to a standing position as you exhale.

TREADING
Standing in shoulder-deep water, bicycle with your legs and scull with your hands, palms down. You may hold the side of the pool with one hand for balance, if necessary.

FLUTTER KICKING
Hold onto the side of the pool while lying on your stomach in the water. Do a flutter kick by kicking your legs into a horizontal position while keeping your knees straight. Move each leg alternately up and down in rapid succession. Extend elbows as far as possible.

CLIMBING
Stand in the water and hold onto the side of the pool with both hands. Place your feet against the side of the pool. Walk up and down the side.

KNEE FLEXION
Hold onto the side while lying on your back in the water. Bring knees up to chest. Hold for 5 seconds before extending your knees.

RUNNING IN PLACE
Stand in chest-deep water and run in place. Maintain balance by placing hands palms down in the water, with elbows flexed 90 degrees.

PULL-UPS
Place arms on the edge of the pool. Raise body weight until arms are extended, then lower in controlled movement.

LEG LIFTS
With your back against the side of the pool wall, tuck knees to chest, then slowly lower knees.

BICYCLE KICKS
Lie on your back in the water, holding onto the pool side. Pull one knee into your chest as you extend the other leg. Alternate legs.

Remember that the pace of exercise is determined by level of fitness. Those who are unfit will have to work relatively hard just to move around. As fitness improves, more strenuous activity is possible. This means that although two people are working at a completely different pace, each may be working just as hard. This is why it is important to do aerobic activity with people of a similar fitness level or to have an instructor who knows how to run a class with participants of varying fitness levels.

There are many types of aerobic activity, including:
• Walking
• Swimming
• Jogging
• Cycling
• Water aerobics
• Cross-country skiing

- Rope skipping
- Aerobics classes, which vary in difficulty and quality. Always be sure to get a qualified instructor who is concerned that participants exercise appropriately.
- Step aerobics, which involve the use of a step to increase difficulty of the workout
- Low-impact aerobics, using exercises that minimize the stress on joints

Note: In an aerobics class (or any other fitness class), you are the ultimate judge of how strenuous the exercise needs to be. If you feel you are working too hard, don't let anyone talk you out of easing up or stopping completely, if necessary.

Duration

An aerobic exercise session should last 20 to 30 minutes. Some evidence suggests that one can break this down into small segments. For example, instead of walking for 30 minutes, walk three times for 10 minutes. This is more of a practical matter. If you can exercise for the allotted time all at once, we encourage you to do that; it is more likely that you will get the exercise done. It is comforting to know, however, that even if you do not have a block of time, breaking exercise down into smaller segments is effective, too.

Frequency

Plan to do aerobic exercise three to five times a week.

Training effect

You can improve aerobic capacity by increasing the amount of time spent exercising or increasing the pace. With continued aerobic workouts, your heart rate will not get as high while working out at the initial level, and harder work (e.g., walking faster and/or longer) will be easier to tolerate. Your resting heart rate will also be reduced.

Resistance exercise

Resistance exercises, in which you train against a resisting force, are essential for developing strength and for developing and preserving lean muscle mass—the force that drives metabolism. Strong muscles are also important for the smooth and easy performance of everyday activities such as carrying groceries (mainly fruit and vegetables, of course!), lifting boxes, and walking up stairs.

To perform resistance exercise, you may lift weights (using free weights or machines) or perform aqua exercises in which water provides the resistance.

The two elements of resistance exercises that provide a training effect are:
- The degree of resistance (how heavy the weight is)
- The number of repetitions or "reps" (how many times you lift the weight)

As you practice resistance exercises, your strength and endurance improve and the weight and/or the number of repetitions can be increased. You do not have to be a bodybuilder to get benefits from resistance training. Resistance exercises help strengthen bone and prevent it from becoming brittle. Because of this, resistance exercises, typically a routine with hand-held weights, are essential for women who are especially at risk for bone degeneration disorders like osteoporosis. Resistance exercises are also important for older people, because preserving bone and muscle substantially improves the quality of life.

Rules of Resistance Exercise

Always warm up with simple stretching.

Work slowly.

Keep breathing while doing the exercise. (There is a tendency to hold your breath while lifting a weight.)

Do not work beyond the point of mild discomfort.

Stop if you feel any pain.

Cool down by repeating your warm-up stretching routine.

Guidelines for Lifting Weights

By adjusting the amount of weight lifted and the number of repetitions performed, weight training can emphasize either muscle strength or endurance. Heavy resistance with few repetitions works best for developing strength. Light resistance with many repetitions is the key to developing endurance.

Duration

Start with a weight that you can lift comfortably for six repetitions. When you can comfortably do ten repetitions, switch to a higher weight.

A good resistance program involves working each of the major muscle groups at least once during a workout. When working on the same muscle group with consecutive exercises, rest for at least 2 minutes between exercises to allow the muscles to recover. A resistance program can be completed in 20 to 30 minutes. Suggested routines appear at the end of this chapter; Series B and Series C sessions include resistance exercises.

Frequency

Do your resistance workout three times a week, with at least one day off between sessions. This allows the muscles to recover and avoids straining and overexertion.

Training effect

As you continue resistance exercises, the size and weight of your muscles will increase. It will be easier for you to lift the initial weight.

Flexibility exercise

Flexibility exercises tone muscle and keep it supple. They also help develop better muscular and body control. There are various types of flexibility/stretching exercises, including yoga.

Duration

Start by holding a stretch for 10 seconds. With practice, you can comfortably hold a stretch for up to 60 seconds. Never stretch beyond the point of comfort.

Frequency

Do your flexibility workout every day.

Training effect

Improved muscle tone and body control will result from regular flexibility exercise. Stretching exercises appear at the end of this chapter in the Series A session.

Calculating caloric expenditure

The following table will give you an idea of the energy expenditure for certain activities. These figures are approximations that will differ, depending on the person's metabolic rate.

Calories Burned by Various Activities

Calories burned/hour	Activity
70 to 85	Sitting
100 to 240	Typing/office work
150 to 250	Gardening/yard work
250 to 300	Bowling Walking 3 mph Ballroom dancing Mowing the lawn
300 to 350	Table tennis Volleyball Doubles tennis
350 to 400	Walking 4 mph Chopping wood Shoveling snow
400 to 450	Walking 5 mph Singles tennis Scrubbing floors Cleaning windows

The three principles of fitness

To develop an effective fitness program, you must consider three principles.

• *Specificity.* You need specific exercises to get particular benefits. For instance, aerobic exercises help develop healthier heart and lungs. No single exercise can give you a complete workout.

• *Overload.* The body adapts when it is faced with manageable overload. To improve fitness, the overload needs to be slowly but progressively increased. The three dimensions of overload are:
  1. *Frequency*: how often the exercise is performed (typically three times a week).
  2. *Intensity*: how difficult the exercise is.
  3. *Duration*: how long the exercise is performed.

• *Reversibility.* The body adapts to the demands placed on it. Sensible workout techniques, practiced regularly, will improve fitness. Fitness will decrease if those exercise routines are not maintained.

Designing your own exercise program

In designing an effective program, focus on three specific areas: assessment, goal setting, and choosing activities. In the next section, action steps will help you get started.

An assessment of current fitness levels will allow you to determine exercise goals and monitor progress. It does not matter what level you start at—improvement will come once you have developed an exercise routine.

There are three basic categories of fitness:

1. *Cardiorespiratory endurance*: the ability to perform moderately strenuous activity over an extended period of time

2. *Muscular strength and endurance*: the ability to exert a maximum force and repeat an action or hold a position for an extended period of time

3. *Flexibility*: the ability to move a joint through its range of motion

Aerobic/cardiorespiratory exercise
Assessment
The simplest way to assess your cardiorespiratory endurance is to perform a 3-minute step test. In this test, you step up and down on a bench, a stack of firmly-tied newspapers, or some other solid object 12 inches high. A cycle consists of stepping onto the bench with one foot, bringing the other foot up to the bench, then stepping back to the floor. You may alternate which foot steps first. Do twenty-four cycles per minute for 3 minutes. Stop after 3 minutes and immediately count your pulse for 1 minute.

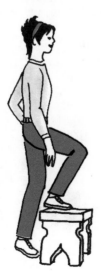

Do this by placing your index, middle, and ring fingers on the underside of your wrist or on your neck (next to the Adam's apple, in the groove between the windpipe and the neck muscle).

Compare your resting heart rate to the chart at the end of this chapter.

Goals
Use your performance on the assessment test to set goals for aerobic activity.

Choice
Although walking is likely to be your aerobic activity of choice, consider other activities that you could use from time to time for variety. Any continuous activity which uses large muscle groups is aerobic. Varying your exercise is important—if nothing else, it prevents boredom.

When beginning an exercise regimen, plan an aerobic activity 3 days a week, gradually increasing to five times a week.

It is helpful to vary the intensity and duration of the training. For example, on some days you might walk 2 miles at a fast pace, and on others 3 miles at a moderate pace.

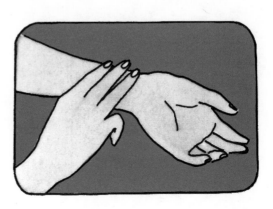

Now, schedule your aerobic activity. Decide what time of the day will work best.

I will do my aerobic exercise on (choose three days)

_____

_____

_____

*At (time of day)*_____

_____

_____

The best time of day for aerobic exercise is the time that you are most likely do it.

Location _____

_____

_____

_____

Muscular strength and endurance
Assessment
To assess muscular *strength*, perform these tests.

Upper body strength
Push-up: Do as many push-ups as you can. You may do the modified version on your knees, keeping the back straight. There is no time limit, but you should do the push-ups continuously with no pausing.

15 to 25 ....Great
5 to 14 ....Average
fewer than 5 ....Need work

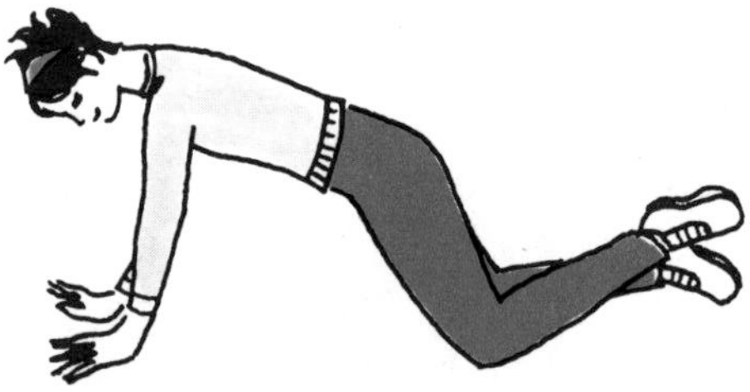

Middle body strength
Abdominal hold: Lie flat on your back with knees bent and heels about 12 inches from the buttocks. Fold your arms across your chest and curl up to a 45-degree angle and hold for as long as you can.

15 to 25 seconds ....Great
5 to 14 seconds ....Average
less than 5 seconds ....Need work

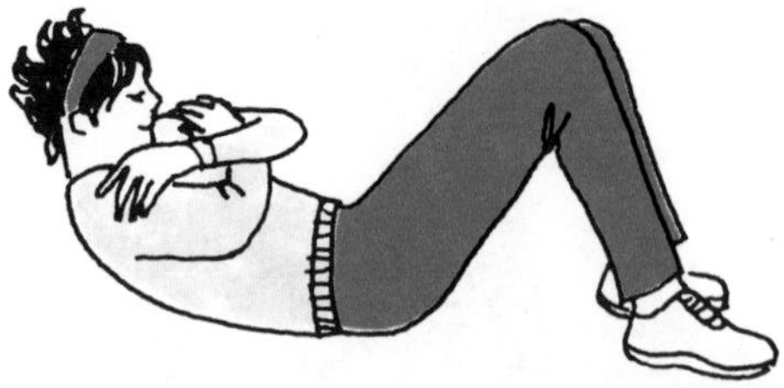

Lower body strength
Wall sit: Lean your back against a wall and bend your legs at a 90-degree angle. Hold for as long as you can.

60 to 90 seconds ....Great
30 to 60 seconds ....Average
less than 30 seconds ....Need work

To assess muscular *endurance*, count the maximum number of contraction repetitions you can do (for example, push-ups or sit-ups) or the maximum time you can hold a muscle contraction (for example, a bicep curl).

Goal
The goal of a complete muscular strength program is to work all the major muscle groups, including upper back, shoulders, arms, chest, abdomen, lower back, thighs, buttocks, and calves.

As a guide to resistance exercises, build *strength* rapidly by working with weights of up to 80 percent of your maximum capacity. For example, if the heaviest weight you can lift is 10 pounds, a good starting weight would be 8 pounds.

For muscular *endurance*, use a weight of 40 to 60 percent of your maximum capacity—for instance, 4 to 6 pounds if the maximum weight you can lift is 10 pounds. As strength increases, use heavier weights.

To improve fitness, you must perform enough repetitions to fatigue your muscles.

Repetitions

Using a *heavy* weight and performing a *low* number of reps (three to six) builds **strength.**

Using a *light* weight and performing a *high* number of reps (fifteen to twenty) builds **endurance.**

For **general fitness,** do eight to twelve reps of an exercise.

Choice
To begin your strength program, choose a weight that you can easily move through six reps for one set. A "set" is a group of repetitions of an exercise followed by a rest period. Gradually add weights and sets until you can perform three sets of ten reps. If you can do more than twelve reps, increase the weight until you can do only seven or eight.

Do these exercises 2 to 4 days a week. Always allow a day of rest between workouts to let muscles recover.

You will notice an increase in strength soon after starting these exercises. Changes in muscle size begin after 6 to 8 weeks.

Now, schedule your strength and endurance activity.

I will do my strength and endurance exercise on (choose three days)

_____

_____

_____

*At (time of day)*_____

_____

The best time of day for a strength workout is the time that you are most likely do it.

Location _____

_____

_____

Flexibility

Assessment

To assess flexibility, try these tests.

Sit and reach: This test measures muscle flexibility in your lower back and in the back of your legs. Good leg and back flexibility help you avoid lower back pain as well as back and leg injuries.

Sit on the floor with your legs extended in front of you, heels about six inches apart, soles of your feet touching a wall. Without bending your knees, reach forward as far as possible at toe height, attempting to touch the wall and bringing your forehead as close to your knees as possible. Do not jerk forward; move your body only until you feel a slight tug. Hold that position and imagine the muscles relaxing. As you relax, stretch a bit farther until you feel

another tug. Hold for a few seconds and see how far you have reached.

Palms against the wall........Great
Knuckles touch the wall.....Good
Fingertips touch the wall....Average
Fingertips are a
    few inches from toes ....Need work

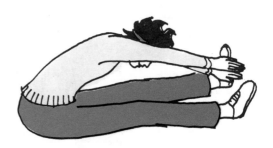

Standing toe touch: This one lets gravity help you a bit! It rates the flexibility of your hamstrings.

Stand with legs straight and feet about shoulder width apart. Tuck your chin to your chest and slowly roll down with arms extended. Keep the hands close to the body; do not reach away from the body. If you can touch your fingertips to the floor, you passed!

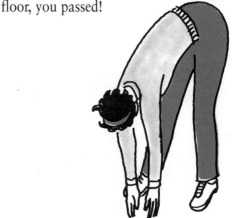

Side stretch: This tests the flexibility of the sides of the body.

Stand with your feet shoulder width apart. Slide your right hand down the side of your leg as you bend to the right. Then try this to the left side. Can you get your hand past your knee?

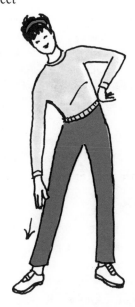

Back clasp: This tests shoulder flexibility.

Sitting or standing, reach over one shoulder with one arm while reaching behind the back with the other arm, and try to grasp hands. Try on both sides.

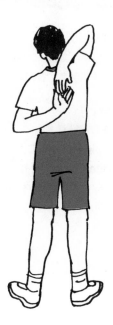

Your hands reach ....Great
  Your hands don't
    quite reach ....Average
  Not even close ....Need work

If your shoulder flexibility needs work, try performing this motion while clasping a towel or other object in both hands.

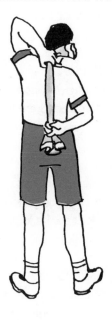

Goal
The goal of exercises in this area is to increase overall flexibility.

Choice
In static stretching, a muscle is stretched gradually, and the stretch is held for 10 to 60 seconds. This slow movement helps you to safely stretch farther than usual. Avoid ballistic stretching, in which muscles are suddenly stretched in a bouncing motion; this can cause injury.

For each static stretch, slowly stretch to the point of slight tension, then hold the position for 10 to 60 seconds. As the tension subsides, stretch a little bit farther. Rest for 30 to 60 seconds. Repeat each stretch three to five times.

A complete flexibility workout will take between 15 and 30 minutes. Do a flexibility workout three to five times a week, especially after a workout when your muscles are warm.

What to Look for in a Walking Shoe

UPPER
Leather or leather and mesh are best for breathability and wear.

TOE BOX
Should give toes enough room to wiggle and protect them from stubbing. Some shoes have a toe "wrap" for extra protection.

OUTER SOLE
Durable rubber provides stability and traction. Look for flexibility across the ball of the foot so the foot can bend naturally as you walk.

ANKLE COLLAR
The collar is padded for comfort and secure fit. Sometimes it is notched in the back to support the Achilles tendon.

INSOLE
A pliable liner, usually removable, provides extra cushioning.

TONGUE
Should be padded and fit securely under laces without sliding.

ARCH
An internal rubber arch cushion adds support. Snug fit helps prevent foot fatigue.

MIDSOLE
This is the main cushioning and shock-absorbing part of a shoe, so it must be well-constructed.

HEEL COUNTER
A hard, cuplike device inside the shoe stabilizes the heel and prevents it from slipping.

Selecting a Health Club or Fitness Facility

KNOW WHAT YOU WANT.
Some clubs focus on group instruction, others on the individual exerciser. Some cater to weight-lifters, others to aerobic dancers.

VISIT THE CLUB.
Visit at the time of day you would use the facility so you can note the classes, clientele, and level of crowding. Is the equipment in good working order? Are exercise areas well-lit, roomy, and ventilated? Instructors should be certified through an accredited organization.

ASK ABOUT MEMBERSHIP TERMS.
Some clubs have reciprocal arrangements with other facilities. Is there a trial membership?

LOOK FOR AN ESTABLISHED FACILITY.
The health club industry is fickle. You may sign up for a club that could close without refunding money to members. Read the contract carefully.

Now, schedule your flexibility workout.

*I will do my flexibility exercise on
(choose three days)*

_____

_____

_____

*At (time of day)*_____

_____

The best time of day for a flexibility workout is the time that you are most likely do it.

Location _____

_____

_____

Good exercise practices
Warming up and cooling down

It is essential that you prepare for both
starting and stopping exercise, especially
aerobic exercise. You must make a smooth
transition from a resting to an active state
and vice versa. Suddenly starting or stopping vigorous activity can be a shock to
the system and may lead to problems.

Warming up consists of two components.

1. *Stretch* to loosen muscles and prepare
   physically and mentally for the upcoming exercise. Simple stretches include
   those of the neck, shoulders, hamstrings,
   and calves. Take about 5 minutes to
   perform these warm-up stretches.

2. *Start slowly.* Do the first phase of exercise
   at a slower pace to gradually get lungs
   and heart used to an increased workload.

Cooling down consists of the same two
principles. Toward the end of your exercise period, enter a cool-down phase by
slowing gradually. When finished, stretch
your muscles. You gain maximum benefit
by stretching when muscles are warm, so
this is a great time for a short stretch routine. Again, work all the major muscle
groups. By the end of the cool-down
period, your body should have returned
to normal, with heart rate, breathing, and
circulation restored almost to pre-exercise
levels. One indication of fitness is how
quickly pre-exercise heart rate levels are
restored after working out.

Common questions about exercise

Is exercise safe for me?
If you have any questions about your
health, consult your doctor before beginning, continuing, or increasing exercise.
Generally speaking, there are almost
always some exercises that can be performed safely, but knowing exactly what
they are and how and when to do them
requires expert input.

*Okay, but are there any times when I definitely
should not exercise?*
If you are injured, you should not exercise
without first checking with a physician or
a sports medicine specialist. Also, do not
exercise if you have a fever.

What kind of clothing should I wear?
Workout clothes should feel comfortable,
allow free movement, and let the body

cool itself. Footwear is especially important. Wear shoes that are appropriate for the activity. When walking, wear a good pair of walking shoes (not tennis shoes or cheap sneakers). When jogging, wear a good pair of jogging shoes (not tennis shoes or cheap sneakers). For general aerobic activity, wear cross-training shoes (not tennis shoes or cheap sneakers). When playing tennis, wear tennis shoes (not cheap sneakers).

Should I work out with other people?
If working out with others makes it more likely that you will do your exercise, then by all means work out with *supportive* people who are at the *same fitness level* as you. Many people prefer to work out alone, and this is perfectly acceptable. Just do whatever makes it more likely that you will exercise.

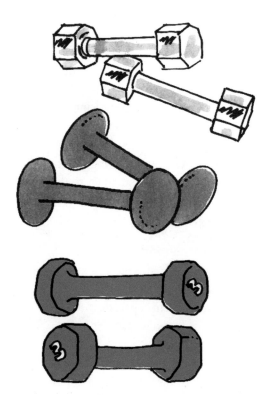

Treatment of Minor Exercise Injuries: The RICE Method

To recall the steps in proper treatment of minor injuries, just think of the initials R-I-C-E.

REST:
Stop using the injured area as soon as you feel pain.

ICE:
Immediately apply ice to the injured area for 15 to 20 minutes. Reapply ice several times a day for 48 hours after injury occurs (or until swelling disappears). Don't have an ice pack? Use a bag of frozen vegetables—it molds well to the affected body part.

COMPRESSION:
Wrap the injured body part with an elastic bandage to minimize swelling.

ELEVATION:
Raise the injured part above heart level to decrease blood supply to the area.

Note: Heating pads or analgesic rubbing creams do not help heal exercise injuries.

Get medical attention if you suspect possible ligament injuries or broken bones, or if you experience internal disorders such as chest pain, fainting, and heat reactions. Injuries that don't heal within a reasonable amount of time also need medical attention.

How does exercise affect my body composition?
Aerobic exercise burns calories, helping to create a negative energy balance and reduce fat. Weight training increases lean body mass and helps preserve, and even build, muscle. By increasing metabolism, weight training also contributes to fat loss.

Should I invest in exercise equipment?
Indoor exercise equipment can be very useful, especially if you live in a climate in which it's often too hot or too cold to exercise outside. Here are some guidelines for the purchase of exercise equipment.

• Choose equipment that reflects your natural preferences. If you are a walker, invest in a treadmill. Ski machines are for skiers, rowing machines for rowers.

• Buy the best equipment you can afford. The power of the machine is important; make sure it's powered by a good belt. Basically, you get what you pay for.

• Only invest in a piece of equipment if you are sure you are going to use it. Thousands of treadmills and other pieces of equipment currently serve as nice clothes racks.

How can I avoid injuries?
Nearly one-third of exercisers abandon their programs because they get injured. Most of these are minor injuries, but even a minor injury can throw you off schedule, and you may never resume your routine. Avoid injuries by:

• *Exercising regularly.* Develop a regular routine. Sporadic exercisers are more likely to get injured.

• *Using proper equipment.* Never use equipment, or perform any exercise, if you are unsure of how to do properly.

• *Always warming up and cooling down appropriately.* You significantly reduce the risk of injury by following this simple rule.

• *Wearing appropriate footwear* (not cheap sneakers).

• *Not overdoing either the intensity or frequency.* Stay within what is possible.

• *Seeking professional treatment for injuries* before they become problems.

• *Listening to your body.* You know what is realistic.

What can I do if I hate exercise?
You need to accept that successful weight management requires regular physical activity. There are things that you can do, however, to make exercise more enjoyable. Most exercise, especially aerobic exercise like walking and biking, does not require you to pay attention to the exercise per se. Most people already know how to walk. The key is occupying your mind with fun thoughts while exercising. Things that you can do include:

• Exercise with a TOPS friend.

• Listen to music or books on tape.

• If exercising indoors (on a treadmill, for example), read, or watch television or videos. You could even talk on the phone.

• Daydream. Movement is conducive to daydreaming. Fantasizing and daydreaming are important creative activities for which adults often don't allow enough time. Exercise provides wonderful opportunity to let creative juices flow.

Almost any activity, including exercise, can be made enjoyable if the mind is entertained.

Walking Schedule

Beginning Level

Step	Minutes walking	Total time in minutes
1	5	5
2	7	7
3	9	9
4	11	11

Intermediate Level

Step	Warm-up	Training pace	Cool-down	Total time
5	3 min	5 min	3 min	11 min
6	3	7	3	13
7	3	9	3	15
8	3	11	3	17
9	4	12	4	20
10	4	16	4	24
11	4	20	4	28
12	4	24	4	32
13	5	26	5	36
14	5	30	5	40

How can I keep my exercise going?
It is very important to plan exercise in advance rather than just "winging it" on a daily basis. Exercise needs to be built into your schedule.

Don't just put exercise in a journal/appointment book, but see exercise as an important investment of time. It is a very important appointment that must not be broken.

If for some reason there really is no time to exercise, try to do some activity, even if it's just for 5 minutes. *Preserving your routine is critical.*

If you happen to get off track, resume as soon as possible with minimal goals. Don't set yourself up for failure. Just aim to get back into a routine.

Walking program

Walking uses large muscle groups that are essential for fitness. It is rhythmic, self-pacing, and safe. Walking at speeds of 4 to 5 miles per hour can burn about 100 calories or more per mile.

The following is a general description of a starter walking program. First, aim to walk 3 days a week. As you progress, your program will be broken down into three stages as follows:

1. *Warm-up*: simple stretches followed by 3 to 5 minutes of slow-paced walking
2. *Training*: 5 to 30 minutes of moderate-paced walking
3. *Cool-down*: 3 to 5 minutes of slow-paced walking followed by simple stretches

It is not necessary to do very strenuous, high-intensity exercise to derive benefits from walking. You just need to maintain a moderate effort continuously for several minutes. If you go more than 3 days without walking, back up one step in the schedule.

Initially, you should progress by increasing your walking time rather than by walking faster.

Walk half of the total time before turning around and returning to your starting point. When you are almost back to the starting point, ask yourself *How do I feel?* and *How much work is this for me?* and *Could I comfortably do more?* If the answers to these questions are *I feel strong,*

This is fairly easy, and *I could comfortably do more,* then move to the next step for your next walk. On the other hand, if the answers are *I am tired, This feels like work,* and *I need to rest,* then remain at the same step for your next walk.

You should increase your walking time every time you walk unless the answers to the questions dictate that you stay at the same step. This will help you increase your rate at the right pace.

Right now, your goal is to increase the time you spend walking and not the pace at which you walk. Pace will become more important after you have reached step 14 in the chart on page 84. Increase your pace gradually and comfortably until you are able to walk the total time with no difficulty.

An exercise quiz

1) Why is lean muscle mass important in weight loss?
2) What must you do before each exercise session?
3) Which of these activities is not an aerobic activity? a) walking b) vacuuming c) swimming d) lifting weights
4) True or false? Cheap sneakers are acceptable footwear for any exercise.

Answers:
1) It increases the rate of metabolism.
2) Warm up
3) d–lifting weights
4) False

The following exercise routines will help you improve and maintain your strength and flexibility. For suggestions on how to incorporate these routines into your daily life, see the 28-day guide starting on page 135.

Series A: Sessions 1-10

A-1
Arm Circles
Do full, slow, sweeping circles with both arms. Circle arms forward, then backward. Exhale as arms come down.

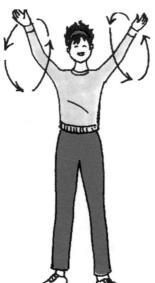

A-2
Side Stretch
Reach one arm down the outside of the leg while exhaling. Hold. Repeat on other side.

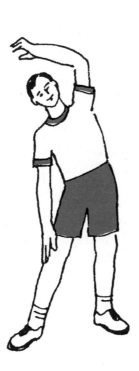

A-3
Trunk Twists
Twist trunk gently to one side, reaching the arm behind and bending the other arm across the stomach while exhaling. (Let the arms "flap" against the sides.) Repeat on the other side.

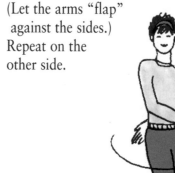

A-4
Sit and Reach
Sit with one leg bent, sole of foot near knee of the straight leg. Gently curl upper body toward knee of straight leg and reach hands forward while exhaling. Hold. Do not bounce. Relax, then repeat. Change leg positions and repeat on other side.

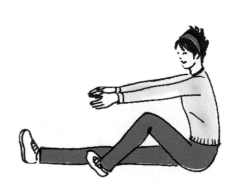

A-5
Single Knee Press
Lie on back. Gently grasp hands behind one knee and bring knee toward chest while exhaling. Hold. Return to starting position and repeat alternately with other leg.

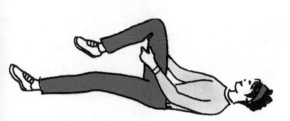

A-7
Peek-Ups
Lie on back, knees bent, feet flat on floor. Lift head and shoulders off floor and look toward knees while exhaling. Relax. Repeat.

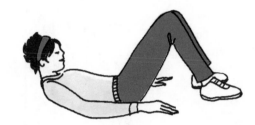

A-6
Mad Cat
On all fours, arch, tucking chin to chest and exhaling. Hold the position, but don't hold your breath. Relax, returning to "flat back" position. Don't sag.

A-8
Prone Stretch
Lie on stomach, arms outstretched in front, resting on the floor. Leaving them on the floor, slide left arm forward and push left foot back while exhaling. Hold. Relax. Repeat with the right arm and right foot.

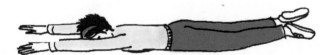

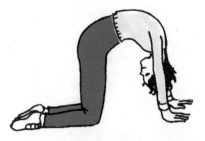

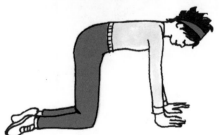

A-9
Wall Push-Offs

Stand flatfooted, facing a wall from a distance of about 2 feet. Starting with arms fully extended, lean into the wall, keeping entire body straight and feet flat on the floor. Then push off from the wall until arms are fully extended. Lower yourself back into the wall.

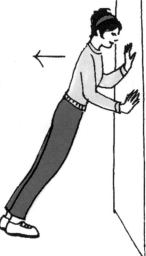

A-10
Neck Stretches

Sit or stand upright, arms and shoulders relaxed. Slowly let head tilt toward right shoulder, then left. Use a continuous relaxed motion. Don't hunch shoulders.

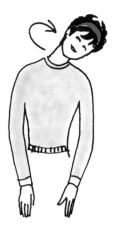

Series B: Sessions 11-20
B-1
Double Knee Press

Lie on back, legs bent, feet flat on floor. Pull knees to chest, grasping backs of thighs while exhaling. Return to starting position, then repeat.

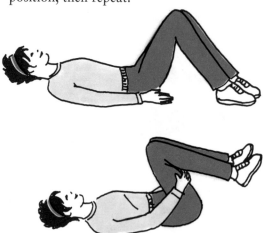

B-2
Chest Stretch

Stand in a corner with forearms on wall. Lean chest to wall. (You should feel this stretch in the chest and near the armpits.) Hold for five counts. Repeat five times.

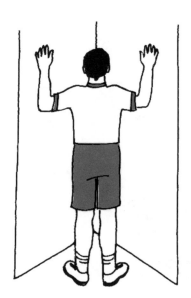

B-3
Toe Raises

Stand with balls of feet on a step so that heels are 2 to 3 inches off the floor. Lower heels below step level, then lift heels a few inches above the step.

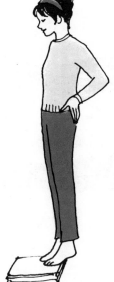

B-4
Wall Squat

Lean against a wall and bend your knees as though you were sitting in a chair. Support your weight with your legs. Begin by holding position for 5 to 10 seconds. Build up to a minute or more.

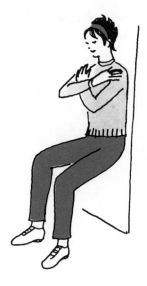

B-5
Press-Up

Lie face down with hands next to armpits. Slowly push yourself up until your upper body is resting on your forearms. Relax and hold for 5 to 10 seconds. Gradually progress to straightening your elbows while keeping your hip bones on the floor.

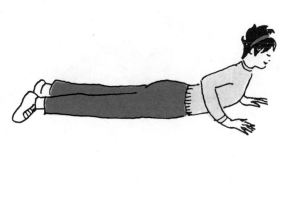

B-6
Leg Curl and Stretch

On all fours in a kneeling position, curl one knee in toward nose while exhaling, then slowly extend leg backward to horizontal position with leg straight. Relax, then repeat with other leg.

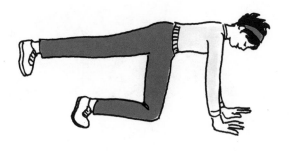

B-7

Lying Bicycle Ride

Lie on your back, hands behind head, knees bent. Pull right knee up toward your chest as you angle the left elbow toward the right knee, twisting upper body. Alternate sides. Move at a smooth, steady pace.

B-9

Swimming

Lie face down. Do front crawl stroke motion, first with one arm, then the other, swinging arms over top.

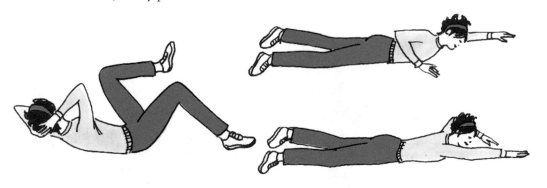

B-8

Chair Dips

Begin by squatting in front of a sturdy chair or low coffee table. Place hands on the front edge with fingers pointing toward your hips. Bend elbows and lower hips toward the floor as low as possible. Push yourself back up until arms are straight. Repeat.

B-10

Knee Lifts

Sit on a sturdy chair, holding the edge for support. Raise bent knees to chest, then slowly return feet to the floor.

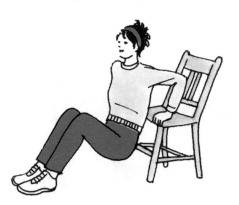

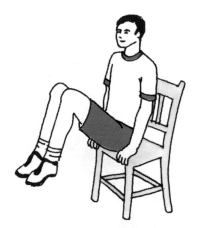

Series C: Sessions 21-30

C-1
Arm Crossovers
Hold arms outstretched
near shoulder height.
Cross them
in front while
exhaling, then
slowly swing
them behind.

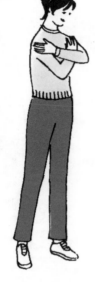

C-3
Leg Lunges
Stand with feet close together. Take a big
step forward and lower yourself into a
lunge position, keeping
back straight. Push
yourself back into the
starting position and
repeat with the other
leg. Build up to three
sets of ten repetitions
on each leg. Once you
achieve this level,
you can add hand
weights to your
routine.

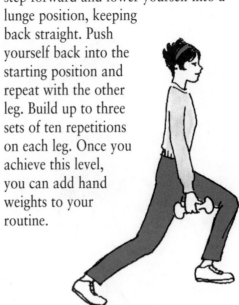

C-2
Chair Crunch
Place legs on a chair with knees bent at a
90-degree angle. With arms crossed in
front or extended at sides, lift head and
shoulders off the floor. Do not use
momentum to come up; let abdominal
muscles do the work.

C-4
Chest Press
Lie on your back with weights in each
hand (using an overhand grip), hands
slightly wider than shoulder width apart.
Press the weights up to an extended position as you exhale. Lower them down to
mid-chest as you inhale. Be sure to use
strict form in this movement and concentrate on pushing with the chest muscles.

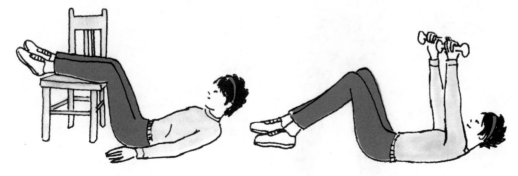

C-5

Bicep Curls

Hold weights in each hand. Stand with feet comfortably apart, elbows close to your sides. Slowly curl one weight up to your chin, turning your thumb away from your shoulder. Lower the weight back to your side and repeat with the other arm.

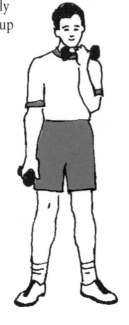

C-6

Tricep Extension

Stand with feet comfortably apart. Hold light weight in one hand. Raise weight to overhead position. Gradually lower the weight behind yourself to base of neck; pause. Push the weight back to the starting position. Work up to eight to ten repetitions on each arm. It's important to keep your elbow behind your head throughout this exercise. If you prefer, do this exercise seated.

C-7

Shoulder Shrugs

Stand with feet comfortably apart. Hold a weight in each hand. Drop chin toward chest to avoid straining the neck. Shrug shoulders up toward ears, pause, and roll shoulders back and downward to starting position.

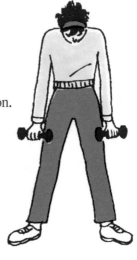

C-8

Side Leg Raise

Lie on one side, using your top hand to prop yourself up so you remain in position. Lift top leg slightly higher than hip level. Gently pulse up the top leg without rotating it, keeping foot parallel to the floor. Work up to fifteen to twenty repetitions on each leg. To add resistance, wear heavy skiing or hiking boots!

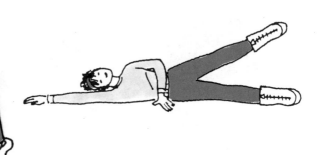

C-9

Pelvic Tilt

Lie on back with feet about 12 inches apart
and soles flat on the floor. Arms should be
out to the sides for support. Tilt pelvis up
toward the ceiling and raise hips a few inches
off the floor. Tighten gluteal (buttocks) and
abdominal muscles and hold for five to ten
counts. Do not arch the back; try to keep it
flat against the floor. Pelvic tilts can also be
done while standing or leaning against a wall.

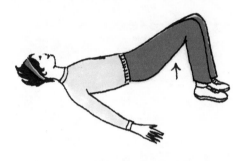

C-10

Flutter Kick

Sit on the edge of a chair, legs straight
out, and alternately kick each one rapidly
as if you were swimming. Work up to
fifty to 100 repetitions.

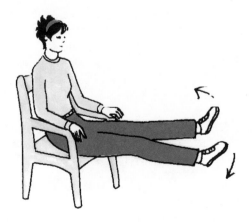

Exercise benefit zones

For optimal benefit, aerobic exercise
should bring your heart rate to between 60
and 85 percent of your maximum heart
rate (MHR) and keep it there during the
aerobic portion of your workout. Start
counting your pulse within 15 seconds of
stopping the exercise (before cooling
down), because heart rate drops significantly upon completion of the exercise.

You can determine your exercise intensity
at any time during your workout. One
method is to check your pulse and use the
exercise benefit zone table on page 94.
This table gives the pulse rates that fall
within the exercise benefit zone for different ages. The pulse rates are given per
minute and per 10 seconds.

Recovery heart rate

To improve cardiorespiratory endurance,
the heart muscle has to be overloaded.
This is accomplished by making the heart
pump more blood and beat faster for a
certain period of time. When the heart
muscle adapts to this overload, it becomes
a stronger, more efficient pump. It beats
fewer times per minute but pumps more
blood with each beat. Not only does resting heart rate decrease, but the time to
revert to recovery rate following exercise
also decreases, an indication of an efficient cardiovascular system.

From time to time, take the 3-minute step
test (described earlier in this chapter) to
see how your heart rate is responding to
aerobic exercise.

Immediately after stopping aerobic exercise,
take a 1-minute pulse to check your recovery heart rate. Consult the recovery heart
rate chart (page 94) for a measure of your
fitness.

Exercise Benefit Zone

AGE	Estimated MHR per minute	60% of estimated MHR		85% of estimated MHR	
		60 SEC.	10 SEC.	60 SEC.	10 SEC.
25	195	117	20	166	28
35	185	111	19	157	26
45	175	105	18	149	25
55	165	99	17	140	24
65	155	93	16	132	22

MHR = Maximum Heart Rate

Recovery Heart Rate–Beats Per Minute

Age	Great	Good	Average	Fair	Not so good
Female 14-29	79 or less	80-101	102-119	120-133	134 and over
30-39	83 or less	84-105	106-122	123-135	136 and over
40-49	87 or less	88-108	109-118	119-130	131 and over
50-59	91 or less	92-113	114-123	124-136	137 and over
60-plus	94 or less	95-117	118-127	128-140	141 and over
Male 14-29	74 or less	75-90	91-100	101-120	121 and over
30-39	77 or less	78-99	100-109	110-125	126 and over
40-49	79 or less	80-100	101-112	113-125	126 and over
50-59	85 or less	86-105	106-115	116-130	131 and over
60-plus	89 or less	90-108	109-118	119-130	131 and over

LIFESTYLE CHOICES & HEALTHY BEHAVIOR

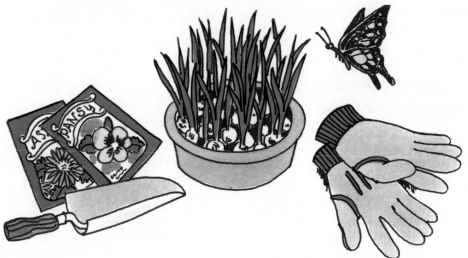

A **weight-management** program does not occur in a vacuum. It needs to take priority, and it requires life-management skills. None of the actions outlined throughout this guide are difficult. You can, and no doubt occasionally do, follow a sensible diet and exercise program. Of course, occasionally following these behaviors is quite different from maintaining them on a regular basis.

This chapter focuses on issues that affect your ability to implement a successful weight-control program:

- Identifying and maintaining your motivation
- Adopting self-management strategies that work for you
- Managing temptation and craving
- Coping with compulsive eating and bingeing
- Managing anger, stress, and frustration
- Dealing with others

Weight management is a lifelong struggle. There will be times when you feel you are really focused on your program and other times when you feel you are completely off track. This is normal in any important project. *The secrets of managing your weight program are to keep in touch with your motivation and to practice damage control when events make it difficult to stay completely on track.*

Motivation (Why am I doing this, anyway?)

The foundation of any behavior is motivation. There are almost as many reasons for wanting to lose weight as there are people trying to do it. Although motivation varies from person to person, some motives will sustain your effort and others will not.

Motives that can keep you on track stem from a desire to improve life in some way. You may want to be healthier, look better, feel younger, wear smaller clothes, or have more energy. All of these outcomes concern the desire for self-improvement. In fact, all legitimate motivation boils down to one concept: *You care enough about yourself to make positive changes.*

Motivation that is not effective involves taking action to please other people. Losing weight to impress your spouse, to make your friends like you, or to appease your children is not likely to succeed in the long run unless it is accompanied by a deep belief that you want these changes for yourself—and that reactions which might or might not occur in other people are a result of your increased self-esteem rather than your decreased clothes size.

Losing weight merely to please other people rarely works because others rarely react the way you think they will once you have lost weight. Even if your weight loss produces a positive response in them, in the end you will resent basing your behavior on the need to please other people (even if you are responsible for this need).

Some years ago, two psychologists, James Prochaska from the University of Rhode Island and Carlos Di Clemente from the University of Texas, suggested a simple five-stage model of motivation:

1. *Precontemplation.* In this stage, through either ignorance or denial, you don't even think about change. Typical thought in the precontemplation stage: "There's nothing wrong with my weight."

2. *Contemplation.* In this stage, you become aware of the problem and begin considering change but do not yet take action. Typical thought in the contemplation stage: "Perhaps I could lose a few pounds, but this isn't the time for me to do it."

3. *Preparedness.* Now you are ready for change and are preparing to take action. Typical thought in the preparedness stage: "I'd better start going to my TOPS chapter meetings."

4. *Action.* Now you are committed to taking steps and beginning a program. Typical thought in the action stage: "Here I am, walking with my chapter's walking team."

5. *Maintenance.* Having established a program, you keep it going. Typical thought in the maintenance stage: "I know this works, and I will keep it going."

The key question, therefore, is: What motivates people to move from one stage to another? What typically gets people moving from ignorance, denial, and procrastination to action is *discomfort*.

People are motivated to change behavior because they want to avoid unpleasant negative consequences. They get a health scare, they get completely frustrated because none of their clothes fit, or they can't do some of their favorite activities. These negative consequences create so much discomfort that they get people to think seriously about change.

What negative consequences did you experience that motivated you to seriously consider losing weight?

The negative consequences that motivated me to lose weight were/are:

1._____

_____

_____

2._____

_____

_____

3._____

_____

_____

The Top Ten Reasons for Starting a Weight-Loss Program

- Diagnosed with illness
- Do not feel good physically
- Unable to fit into clothes
- Lack fitness
- Unable to do certain things
- Feel unattractive
- Feel out of control
- Feel powerless
- Feel like an outcast
- Feel depressed

The problem of motivation— "I don't want to think about that!"

You can probably relate to the fact that discomfort motivates change. Looking in your closet for something to wear, you're completely frustrated at being unable to find anything that fits. You walk across the mall parking lot with your friends and find yourself hopelessly out of breath, huffing and puffing just to keep up. You catch your reflection in the shop window and cringe at what you see.

All of these moments of extreme discomfort are likely to motivate you to do something about your weight. The problem is that they are just that—*moments* of discomfort—and chances are that once the moment has passed, you are no longer uncomfortable. The motivation has slipped through your hands. Because these moments are uncomfortable, you will not want to think about them unless it is unavoidable. However, if you don't focus on the discomfort, you will not be in touch with your motivation.

How to stay focused on your motivation

To prevent motivation from fading in and out, you must somehow capture it and keep it in the forefront of your mind. There are various ways of turning temporary motivation into permanent motivation.

Once you have experienced the health scare, felt disgusted after bingeing, or cringed at your reflection in the mirror, you can't deny these feelings. Once you have had the perception that you are obese, at great health risk, or out of control, you really can't put the genie back in the bottle, as much as you would like to do so. Facing up to the realities of these discomforts will move you from precontemplation to contemplation and from contemplation to action.

To capture this motivation, you must turn these discomforts into tangible reality. Following are several ways to do this.

- *Write it down in a short sentence* such as "I am obese," "I am out of control," "I am killing myself," or "I am depressed."

- *Create an image that captures your discomfort.* For instance, recall the uncomfortable motivating moment, or imagine yourself incapable of getting into any of your clothes or performing any activity.

- *Create an image that captures the positive consequences* of overcoming your problem. Examples:
  — Imagine yourself with a new wardrobe of smaller clothes.
  — Imagine yourself being able to do enjoyable activities.
  — Imagine yourself with more energy.
  — Imagine yourself in control.

- *Find a tangible token of your motivation* such as a piece of jewelry, a TOPS charm, or a wristband.

- *Create a phrase that captures your motivation.* Examples:
  — "I am losing weight to gain control."
  — "Better choices lead to better living."

It is important to keep these images, phrases, and tokens in the forefront of your mind. To do this you need to:

- *Practice your imagery.* Conjuring up an image does not take very long. You can spend a few seconds at various times of the day recalling your images. Doing this just before challenging times is useful for dealing with temptation.

- *Post motivational phrases in prominent places.* Keep these messages in your journal, on the bathroom mirror, or on the refrigerator.

- *Keep motivational tokens with you.* Tokens are a reminder of your commitment. Touching your tokens provides a source of comfort and inspiration.

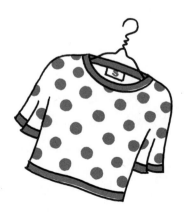

Thoughts on Imagery

Most people can visualize themselves in action.

Some people visualize in color, others do not.

Some see themselves out of their bodies, others in their bodies.

Some visualize in video, some in still-frame.

Some have stronger smell and taste recall than visual recall.

Practice will improve your ability to sense impressions and to conjure up powerful images.

There is a difference between what motivates people to *change* their behavior and what motivates them *to keep the program going* once the changes have been made. Once a weight-control program has been established, motivation begins to change. What motivates people to *maintain* their weight losses?

People are motivated to maintain weight loss not so much by the avoidance of negative consequences but by the positive effects of their success. The reasons people typically give for maintaining their efforts are:

• I feel so much better.
• I have more energy.
• I look better.
• I feel more in control.
• I can do more activities.

If you are a KOPS member in the maintenance phase of your program, what motivates you to continue your weight-control efforts?

I am motivated to maintain my efforts because:

1._____

_____

_____

2._____

_____

_____

3._____

_____

_____

It is important to continue working on the motivational aspect of your program even in the maintenance phase. It is easy to take your progress for granted and get derailed.

Self-management

You cannot achieve anything meaningful in life unless you organize your activity to make that success possible. To do this you need:

• Specific goals
• Good time management
• A monitoring system

Specific goals

The behaviors needed to establish a sensible weight-management program are outlined throughout this book. In the 28-day guide that follows, you will be asked to personalize your goals for health, eating, exercise, and self-care, so that on any given day you know what you are trying to accomplish.

Remember, setting goals is a way of structuring your program. Goals can always be modified at a later date.

Goal-Setting

Goals should be:
- SPECIFIC
  (I will eat *x hundred calories* today.)

- SET WITHIN A TIME FRAME
  (I will eat x hundred calories *today*.)

- MEASURABLE
  (*Did* I eat x hundred calories today?)

- REALISTIC
  (*Can* I eat x hundred calories today?)

Keep your goals prominently displayed in your journal. Review them at the beginning of each day.

Time management—"But how can I fit all of this into my schedule?"

One of the biggest problems many people have with a weight-management program is finding the time to fit in everything necessary to make it work.

To make your weight-loss program a priority, you must find time to accomplish the specific behaviors that make up the program.

For many people, the biggest obstacle is finding the time to exercise. An ideal exercise program requires a minimum of 30 minutes a day, most days of the week. Where is this time going to come from?

- Early morning exercise allows you to incorporate a post-exercise shower into your daily routine, and this works well if you normally shower then anyway.

- You can always break down your aerobic exercise into smaller units of, say, 10 minutes at a time. Thus, you might fit short walking sessions into various times during the day.

- Some stretching and resistance exercises can be done while watching television or doing other activities. So can some aerobic activities, such as those using a treadmill or other indoor equipment.

In the end, you will have to find the time if you want to be successful. This means that you might have to say no to the demands of other people. So before you commit yourself to other activities that may take time away from you and your program, consider the following:
- Always give yourself an opportunity to think before you respond to any request for your time.
- Know where the time is going to come from.
- You can always say no graciously without feeling guilty.
- You will only have yourself to blame if you are overcommitted.

A monitoring system: making sure you get it done

Now that you have established your goals and scheduled your time, let's ensure that you execute your plan.

Even with the best intentions, you will encounter barriers to staying on track: travel, house guests, stress, a faulty alarm clock.

Name five barriers that might prevent you from implementing your program:

1._____

_____

2._____

_____

3._____

_____

4._____

_____

5._____

_____

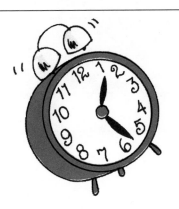

How will you overcome these problems? Write down five ways you could deal with barriers to your program.

1._____

_____

2._____

_____

3._____

_____

4._____

_____

5._____

_____

Keeping track of progress

Awareness of behavior is essential for success. You must track your eating and exercise behavior daily and review it weekly.

A weekly meeting with yourself is necessary to monitor progress, make any necessary modifications, plan goals for the following week, and earn rewards when appropriate. A weekly TOPS weigh-in records progress and provides support and motivation.

Choose one day of the week on which to have your self-management meeting. At this meeting, which need not take very long, you are going to do the following.

- Review your behavior in the past week, paying particular attention to these questions.
  — Did you meet your eating goals?
  — Did you meet your exercise goals?
  — What did you handle well in the past 7 days?
  — What gave you problems?

- If you met your eating and exercise goals, give yourself a reward. Rewards are meant to be tokens of self-appreciation. They should be based on your behavior, not your weight loss. Reward yourself on a short-term basis—that is, once a week where appropriate. Rewards should not consist of food. Examples of appropriate rewards include a visit to a haircutting salon, a new CD or book, a massage, tickets to an event you'd like to attend, or clothing.

- Set your eating and exercise goals for the next week. Since you have your journal in front of you, this is a great time to write down your exercise schedule and eating plans for the next 7 days.

- Plan ahead for any special situations that might occur during the upcoming week. A trip out of town—How are you going to handle that? A big social event—What are you going to do?

- This is also a great time to do any menu planning. You could make a grocery list and schedule your cooking.

Getting yourself organized in this way will really increase your chances of success.

Managing temptations and cravings

Inevitably, temptations and cravings will surface at various points in your life. Learning how to manage these feelings is necessary for long-term success.

First, it is important to understand that cravings are natural and normal. Understand, too, that these feelings can be triggered by a variety of situations or cues.

DID YOU KNOW?
Research shows that food cravings can be triggered by any situation associated with eating.

What situations trigger temptation for you?

1._____

2._____

3._____

4._____

5._____

6._____

7._____

8._____

9._____

10._____

Cravings are often triggered by two types of situations.

The first type is periods when your blood-glucose level is erratic, and especially when the level is declining rapidly. This occurs after consumption of foods high in sugar. Although blood-glucose levels initially increase, they decline quickly, a condition called blood-sugar rebound. This is one reason why small, frequent meals are better than infrequent large ones—blood sugar changes are less erratic. Blood sugar levels also are more erratic during periods of increased hormonal output (e.g., in response to the menstrual cycle or stressful situations). Cravings for sweets are common at these times.

The second trigger for cravings occurs when you face a situation in which you normally eat. Let's suppose it's your habit to eat whenever you get home from work or from running an errand. As you repeat this behavior, your body comes to expect food in this situation. As soon as you put the key in the door, your body gears up for incoming food.

Can I retrain my body?
Yes, it is possible to retrain your body and eliminate many food cravings that are elicited by different situations. The key is that you have to confront the situations associated with this craving and *not eat*.

To continue our example: If you made a concerted effort not to eat when you arrived home, you could break the link between eating and coming home. If you repeated this non-eating pattern enough times, the situation would no longer trigger

temptation. Learning to manage situations that trigger cravings is an important part of managing your weight.

You're telling me I have to confront tempting situations?
Yes, but there are techniques to help you confront temptation. One of the basic premises is: *If you do not feel you can successfully confront temptation, do not put yourself in harm's way.*

Recognize, however, that unless you retreat to your den and become a hermit, you will constantly be faced with tempting situations. A key to this technique is to start slowly with minimal temptation and gradually increase the difficulty as you gain confidence and mastery.

The technique of defusing tempting situations consists of three distinct phases:
1. Imagining yourself successfully resisting temptation
2. Actually resisting moderately tempting situations
3. Actually resisting very tempting situations

Imagining success
Imagery is a powerful weapon in your weight-control effort. Use it to retrain your mind and body to manage temptation. These imagery exercises involve imagining yourself successfully dealing with temptation.

Keep in mind two guidelines for this exercise: Don't practice these imagery exercises when you are hungry, and don't practice them in an environment associated with eating.

Here is a typical imagery practice. First, find a comfortable spot where you will not be disturbed. Turn down the volume on the phones, keep the lights low, and ask anyone else in your immediate environment not to disturb you.

Take a few deep breaths, close your eyes, and imagine the following.

You are at home in the evening watching television, reading, or whatever you are likely to do. There is no one else around. It suddenly occurs to you that ice cream or some other favorite snack would taste good right now. The idea grows that this snack would be really good right now. See yourself going over to where the food is kept. See yourself opening the fridge, freezer, or cupboard. See yourself taking the food out from wherever it is kept. Imagine putting the food down on a table or countertop. It's right there in front of you, ready to eat. You can smell it. You can almost taste it. Focus on that food. There's no one else around. Nobody would know except you. Look again at that food. You can smell it. You can almost taste it. You can almost feel the texture of the food in your mouth. But as you look at the food, you realize how hard you have worked on your program. As you look at that food, you realize that it would taste good for a few seconds but after that you wouldn't feel very good at all. You decide you can do without that food for right now. Imagine yourself throwing the food away. You can hear the whir of the garbage disposal as you throw the food away. As you do, you feel good about being in control.

When encountering this visualization script for the first time, most people balk at the notion of throwing food away. Yet throw-ing food away *in the visualization* is a valuable symbol of control. It is important that you are able to throw food away periodically. It shows that you have detached emotions from food and can see it—even your favorite food—as a disposable commodity. We do not suggest that throwing food away should be an everyday tactic. But it does have great symbolic value, and until you can do it, the food still controls you, not the other way around. *If favorite food exerts a temptation that you find unmanageable, do not have it easily available.*

People object that throwing food away is wasteful. Many people talk about their concern for the starving children of the world. Of course, this is a rationalization. Altering your consumption of food does absolutely nothing to help starving people anywhere in the world. If you really want to help starving people, donate to a reputable charity that fights this problem.

More importantly, the rationalization of not wanting to waste food is tied up with guilt feelings. Many people are trained to feel guilty if they do not eat everything on their plate. There are several reasons why you may want to eat, but guilt should not be one of them.

When you first practice this visualization, it may be difficult to visualize throwing food away or even resisting food. With practice, however, it will become easier to imagine yourself successfully resisting temptation.

Once you have learned how to use this imagery, you can adapt it to your own circumstances. Write down three tempting situations that you could imagine yourself successfully resisting.

1._____

_____

2._____

_____

3._____

_____

These visualizations are critical. They are not only related to managing temptation; they help you develop self-control.

Practice these visualizations regularly. The more you practice, the easier it will be to see yourself coping with temptation. Once you have reached that point, it is time to practice this behavior in real life. You are, of course, constantly faced with temptation, but the next set of exercises encourages you to seek it out! In these exercises, you will confront specific places that create at least a moderate degree of temptation, such as bakeries, ice cream parlors, cookie stores, and food courts.

Write down three such places that are tempting to you.

1._____

_____

2._____

_____

3._____

_____

The next set of exercises calls for you to briefly face these places *without eating*.

For example, go to the cookie store, look at the various cookies, take in the aromas, and leave (quickly, if necessary). Do not eat a cookie. Do not eat anything for at least an hour after this experience. This exercise will retrain your body that the sights and smells of the cookie store are not always followed by eating. *You are practicing the valuable art of resistance.*

With practice, it will be easier to manage not only these specific temptations but temptation in general.

Remember, your best opportunity to develop self-control comes when you are faced with temptation. *Each time you successfully deal with temptation, you are developing your self-control.*

Important tips for managing cravings

• Understand that cravings are often a physical response to specific situations. These feelings are normal and natural. They do not mean that you are unmotivated, lazy, or bad.

• You can handle temptation by changing your response to the situations that trigger it.

• When faced with temptation, realize that the benefits of eating are only short-term—often for only the few seconds that the food is in your mouth.

• Focus on how you will feel if you do indulge. Often, you will regret eating. You might feel depressed and out of control.

• Consider how much effort it takes to burn off the calories you are about to eat. A typical treat provides at least 300 calories, which for most people is the equivalent of about a 3-mile walk.

• Consider how good you will feel if you are able to resist temptation. Realize that you will have strengthened your self-control.

• Disassociate eating with other activities. The more you associate one activity (such as watching TV or reading) with eating, the more that activity will produce the desire to eat.

Cravings are often fleeting. If you can survive the first few seconds of exposure to the food or the tempting situation, it is likely that you will be able to resist it altogether. It is valuable, therefore, to have an automatic first response, an action that will buy you time and prevent automatic eating.

Some automatic first responses include:
• Drink a glass of water or diet soda.
• Physically leave the situation.
• Take ten deep breaths.
• Go brush your teeth.

Write down your automatic first responses:

1._____

_____

2._____

_____

3._____

_____

Remember, if you can survive the first few moments of temptation, there is a good chance that it will fade away.

Bingeing and emotional eating

In the last section you learned how certain situations become associated with eating. This applies to emotions, too. When certain emotions are associated with eating, they can produce a powerful desire to eat. *When you use food to deal with emotions, you are in danger of becoming a binge eater, because any behavior that serves to mask emotions will be done compulsively.*

Millions of people binge. It used to be thought that bingeing was the sole prerogative of the diagnosed bulimic, but we now know that most people who binge do not resort to using laxatives or purging to help control their weight. (To learn more about bulimia, see Chapter 5, Strategies for Special Needs.)

What is a binge?

A binge is difficult to define. Because of cultural and individual differences in eating patterns, it cannot be defined purely in terms of the number of calories eaten. For example, what might be a binge to a ballet dancer or a model may not be a binge to a truck driver or football player.

Bingeing has psychological and biological bases. In addition to learned habits and emotional eating, bingeing can occur as a result of an imbalance of brain chemicals.

Doctors who diagnose mental disorders have recently suggested a new category called binge eating disorder. The criteria for this disorder are:
1. eating more than you want to eat
2. feeling disgusted, guilty, or out of control after the binge

The diagnosis of this disorder requires two binge episodes a week, on average, for the previous 6 months. Men as well as women have binge episodes, although a recent study shows that men are less concerned about the consequences of their bingeing and don't feel as remorseful once they have overindulged.

DID YOU KNOW?
About 35 percent of people on a weight-control program at any one time are diagnosable bingers.

Bingeing typically involves consuming a large number of calories in a short period of time. Because of their physiological and psychological association with comfort, foods high in fat and sugar are the most common choices to comfort or displace difficult emotions. It is not difficult to consume 2,000 calories in a few minutes, and some people have eaten twenty times this amount in a single session.

People who binge usually fall into two overall categories:
1. They are perfectionists who feel that they have to diet perfectly. When they cannot keep up with their own stringent criteria, they abandon all restraint.
2. They use food to mask their feelings.

You don't have to be perfect

One of the problems with a diet is the sense that it is an all-or-nothing proposition—that you are either on the diet or off it. Yet anything as complicated as your eating pattern, anything that dominates so much of your life, anything that involves human behavior, cannot be regulated perfectly all of the time. Human beings, by nature, are imperfect, and you must accept that you are not perfect either.

The secret to success in any human endeavor is perseverance, not perfectionism.

Anything worth doing, especially something as important as getting control of your life, takes effort. There is nothing wrong with trying to manage your program perfectly, as long as you accept that you won't achieve perfection. So the critical question is: What happens when you run into problems?

Perfectionists have a rigid view of the world. Eating 1,000 calories a day is success; eating 1,001 calories is failure. While having some criteria for your performance is admirable, perfectionists treat themselves far too harshly. In fact, they don't give themselves a chance. They set themselves up for failure.

The reasons these traits develop go back to childhood. Children have a natural tendency to accept responsibility for their family dynamics. Children will feel responsible for Dad's drinking, Mom's depression, and Mom and Dad's fights. They will see a connection between their own behavior and these family problems even where none really exists. They will then attempt to make things better through their own behavior, thinking *If I am a good girl, some of these problems will disappear.* Then the child discovers that no matter how hard she tries to be good, the problems don't get better. She concludes that she is not good enough to make it better but persists with the pursuit of perfection, not feeling very good about herself and often considering herself a failure and a disappointment.

Sometimes the child has a fear of success. What if she is perfect but that does not change matters? That means that the child is powerless—not a pleasant thought. Or it means that the adults are out of control—a very scary thought because the child depends on these people for her existence. In that regard, it may be easier to blame herself than to face the fact that her parents, the core of her security and existence, are unstable.

Whatever the dynamics, many people carry around a perfectionist outlook. These people will be great on a program for a few days, then quickly abandon it when they run into a problem. Many are yo-yo dieters who go on and off the diet seeking the perfect answer or despondently giving up any idea of control.

The secret of success on a weight-management program is to accept these truths:
- There is no perfect program or magic solution.
- Anyone will have good days and bad days.
- Perseverance is more important than any other quality.
- Successful weight managers are philosophical about the "off" days and get back on track quickly.

It is unhelpful to beat yourself up about the days you get off track. If you are a perfectionist, you must:
- Accept that deviating from the program does not make you a bad person.
- Realize that having some days when you do not follow the program as you would like is not just normal but inevitable.
- Become more flexible in your thinking.

If you can relax some of your impossibly high standards, you can be successful.

Emotional eating

Using food as a tranquilizer is a common practice. Emotions are powerful, and sometimes it is easier to blot them out with the effects of food rather than face them directly. The use of food to quiet emotions goes right back to infancy, when the crying child is often pacified with food. Sometimes the infant is indeed crying because he is hungry. Sometimes he is crying from distress but gets fed anyway. This can quickly set up the association of food with emotional relief. This association continues as the infant grows. In childhood, food treats are often used to pacify emotions.

The emotions most often associated with food tranquilization are anger, frustration, depression, and a complex of uncomfortable feelings lumped under the title of stress.

Anger, frustration, depression, and stress

Anger
You will feel angry when you believe that you have been treated unfairly. Anger always has a focus; a particular person is responsible for the unfair treatment. Anger is uncomfortable because:

- Physiologically, you feel shaky and hyped up. Anger is often confused with anxiety, and panic attacks are often anger attacks in disguise.

- You fear being out of control. You are never quite sure how angry you might get and whether you will be able to contain yourself.

- Many people are trained to think that anger is wrong. Anger is not a moral issue; it is a basic human emotion.

Many people believe that anger is incompatible with love and that anger means hate. Anger and love are not incompatible. In the course of normal relationships, people close to you are likely to treat you unfairly, and you are likely to be unfair to them. That does not make any of you evil or unloving.

It is important to manage anger by means other than food. Food, specifically high-sugar food, can temporarily block out anger, but this is no answer in the long run.

The steps to effectively manage anger are:

- *Validate anger.* Accept that anger is a normal emotion. Anger is an important act of self-expression. The *management*, not the feeling, of anger is the real issue.

- *Vent anger.* Keeping anger inside can be really uncomfortable, so you need to find acceptable ways of expressing it. Directly addressing the person who is angering you is a good approach but is not always possible. If so, you can express anger by:
  — *Writing it down.* Write that letter (you don't have to send it) or type out those feelings. Don't worry about grammatical style, just get it out!
  — *Talking with somebody.* Find a good, sympathetic listener (not a problem-solver) who will let you vent. If an appropriate friend is not at hand, talk to a professional.
  — *Physically releasing anger through action.* You can burn off extra tension through walking and other aerobic exercise. Use punching bags, pillows, and other hitable objects to express anger.

Imagery exercises are also useful. Imagine yourself letting go of anger as described in the following scenario.

Imagine that you are in a clearing in the woods. In front of you sits a pile of tree limbs and sticks. You are very angry. You are burning inside, red and hot. You start yelling in the direction of the pile of sticks.

As you exhale, you see your red-hot breath carrying the anger out of you. You continue to yell, and you see that the red-hot anger is carried out of you toward the pile of sticks. The pile of sticks catches fire. You stop yelling. You feel much calmer. Standing quietly, you watch the bonfire blaze. You watch from a safe distance until the flames begin to dwindle. Gradually they die out and the fire turns to smoldering ash. Finally it dies completely.

You can also manage anger using other relaxation exercises, such as the deep breathing technique described later in this chapter.

You can use your anger to fuel your weight-control efforts. Don't allow someone else to sabotage your goals. There are too many people walking around wearing their unexpressed anger.

The person who is most affected by your anger is you. Forgiveness will help release you from these potentially destructive feelings.

Frustration
Frustration occurs when you have been thwarted in an attempt to reach a goal. There may not be any one person responsible for this situation—it's just life.

Frustration feels uncomfortable because:
• It is associated with an "antsy" physical state.
• It can interfere with your life plans.
• It may be accompanied by a sense of depression or hopelessness.

Managing frustration involves many of the same techniques described in the management of anger. These include sharing, writing, physical exercise, imagery, and relaxation procedures.

In addition, it may help if you can put frustration into perspective. We never know the real meaning of events until long after they have happened. What may seem like great news now may turn out to be a disaster. Similarly, what may seem like a disaster now may turn out to be a blessing in disguise. Stay philosophical. Life is frustrating. The people who cope best with life are those who are able to deal with adversity and turn it into opportunity.

You can use imagery to manage frustration, too. The exercise below helps you compartmentalize your frustration.

Imagine that you are intensely frustrated. In front of you is a secure box. Lift up the lid and pour all of your frustration into it. Now shut the box and lock it tight. Take the box down to the basement. Find a far corner. Put the locked box in that corner. Push it right up against the wall. After checking to ensure that the box is locked, leave the basement. The box is always there—you know where it is if you need it. Right now, you can keep it out of sight.

Depression
There are many forms of depression. Although depression often accompanies sadness, it is not the same as sadness. Depression involves a loss of energy, and this can happen for a number of reasons. Depression can occur because there is:
• An imbalance in the body chemicals responsible for mood
• A loss, including the loss of a long-time habit
• A lid on the expression of a strong emotion, especially anger
• Fatigue brought about by illness

Symptoms of Depression

• Low energy

• Disturbed sleeping; frequent awakening

• Disturbed eating: loss of appetite in serious cases; increased eating in common depression

• Loss of interest in previously enjoyed activities

• Deterioration of self-care

• Feelings of hopelessness

Depression is a serious and debilitating condition that afflicts millions of people. Fortunately, good treatments are available.

Antidepressants are among the safest and most effective psychoactive medications. They are not addictive, and the newest classes of these drugs have few side effects. The medications most currently used are the *selective serotonin reuptake inhibitors*. These allow more of the important natural chemical serotonin to stay in your brain.

Drugs, however, are just one part of treatment. Counseling aimed at resolving problems and changing thinking patterns is also important. This is true even if you are biologically predisposed to the disorder. It has been shown that cognitive therapy, designed to instill a more positive outlook and help manage the relationship between thoughts, moods, and behavior, is a powerful treatment for depression. Cognitive therapy in combination with anti-depressant medication is the most powerful form of treatment and has helped millions of people.

Stress
There are many different types of stress. The word stress is commonly used to mean at least four different things:
• Time pressure
• Overload
• Traumatic life situations such as illness, relocation, or divorce
• Difficult emotions

People tend to deal with stressful situations by eating more and paying less attention to exercise. Under stress, the body needs more energy, and there is a tendency to get this with a quick fix of sugar. Both sugar and caffeine actually deplete energy, so they are not good choices when you are under stress.

You can take several steps to manage stress.

Exercise. When people undergo stress, their exercise program is the first to suffer. Giving up exercise, however, is abandoning the very activity that can help the most. Exercise will give energy and help relieve tension. Keep some exercise going, even if it is not possible to do your usual routine.

Compartmentalization. Whenever you are in a stressful situation, ensure that there is a way of escaping it, even for a short while. This could mean anything from going to the movies to taking a short trip out of town. Physically removing yourself from the scene of the stress is always helpful.

Relaxation. Taking a 15-minute relaxation break at least once a day is important. The break helps you recharge your batteries and prevents stress and tension from building. There are various relaxation techniques, and they are all beneficial. Find the ones that work for you and practice them on a regular basis, not just when you are under stress.

Activities that promote a state of relaxation include yoga, daydreaming, staring into the fire, meditation, and deep breathing. Simply closing your eyes and resting for 15 minutes can help you get into this state.

Taking a short nap can also be helpful, providing it is only a short nap of no more than 15 minutes. If you sleep too long, you risk interfering with your normal sleep patterns.

Deep Breathing Exercise

- Get into a comfortable position. Have your back well-supported so that you are not slumped; or simply lie down.

- Close your eyes.

- Slowly inhale by taking a deep, controlled breath through your nose.

- Exhale by blowing the air slowly and gently through your mouth.

- As you repeat this, focus on the breath going in and out of your body. Focus on the air going in and out of your lungs.

Meditation Exercise

- Get into a comfortable position in a situation where you will not be disturbed.

- Close your eyes.

- Concentrate on all the different sounds you can hear for 2 minutes.

- When thoughts intrude, don't engage them. Let them pass through your consciousness.

Dealing with others

Other people in your life will influence your weight-control efforts. Many of these people will be well-intentioned but not know how to help you. Others will try to undermine your efforts.

People can have power over you only if you give it to them.

This is your program, and these are your choices. Don't let others interfere with your progress.

It's not possible for other members of your family to be neutral about your weight. Spouses and children are involved if your weight struggles influence your mood and the way you react to loved ones. So, while the choice is yours and the program is yours, it is possible to get your family and friends to help your efforts if they wish to do so.

As with every aspect of a good relationship, communication is the key to getting your family and friends to support you. You can do this by explaining your program to them. Let them know what your goals are and how you are going to achieve them.

Also, show them how they could be supportive. To help you, others need to know what you want. Others could:

• Stop asking how much weight you have lost. Your program involves more than just losing weight. It concerns increasing energy, taking control, and changing behavior.

• Help you make better food choices. They could do this by not offering you high-calorie foods. They could accept that there will be less food in the house, to reduce temptation. They could agree to socialize in functions and at restaurants that are manageable for you.

• Make it more likely that you will exercise. They could mind the kids so you could exercise, or they could offer to exercise with you.

• Encourage you when you are following the program and doing well.

• Encourage you when you are off the program and not doing so well.

You are looking for support, which means anything that will make it more likely that you will stay on the program. You are definitely not looking for:

• Someone to take control and start telling you what to do. This is your program and these are your choices. No one can do it for you.

• Someone feeding you different ideas of how to lose weight. You don't need to hear about hundreds of unrealistic claims and crazy ideas. You know how to lose weight.

• Someone who is negative. Whenever possible, eliminate negative influences from your life. People who tell you what you are doing wrong need to be ignored if they cannot be avoided.

Everyone has his or her own ideas about how to lose weight. Each person must find the elements of a program that are most helpful, but the only one who has the answer to your weight problem is you. The choice is yours!

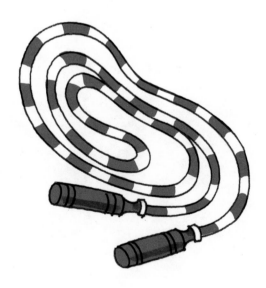

Lifestyle quiz

1) Who has executed their weight
   program to perfection?
2) What are three ways of
   managing stress?
3) If successful, how often should you
   give yourself a reward?
4) How do you get support?
5) What are the five stages of motivation?

Answers:
1) Nobody
2) Exercise, compartmentalization, and
   relaxation
3) Weekly
4) Seek it
5) Precontemplation, contemplation,
   preparedness, action, and maintenance

STRATEGIES FOR SPECIAL NEEDS

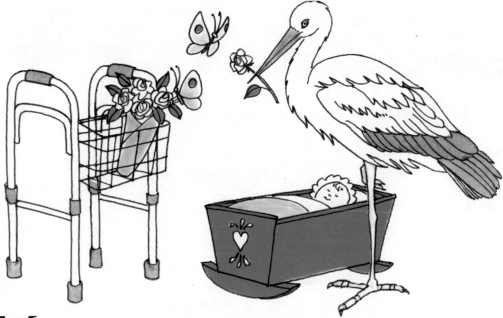

Many people trying to overcome obesity face special challenges that require modifications to a typical weight-loss routine. In this chapter, we will consider these special needs. The first section covers weight-loss strategies for groups with special needs that do not arise from obesity:
- Children and adolescents
- The elderly
- Pregnant and lactating women
- People with hormonal abnormalities
- Menopausal women
- People with limited mobility
- Depressed people

The second section covers the needs of those suffering from illnesses related to obesity or eating patterns:
- Diabetes mellitus
- Hypertension
- Heart disease and stroke
- Gall bladder disease
- Osteoarthritis and gout
- Cancer
- Bulimia

Groups with special needs

Children and adolescents

Obesity among children and adolescents is increasing. The National Health and Nutrition Examination Surveys II and III (NHANES) estimate that over 20 percent of children and adolescents in North America are obese. At puberty, hormones create changes in body composition that typically result in normal self-conscious-ness about body image. These changes accompany the sensitive transition to greater social awareness. Obesity com-pounds these difficult transitions, often diminishing a child's self-esteem, setting up a lifelong concern with body image and linking self-esteem with weight. This is especially true for girls, whose bodies undergo more dramatic and symbolic changes in adolescence.

Obesity in adolescence can create serious social and developmental problems, the more so because they begin at such an early age. Problems associated with obesity in childhood and adolescence include:
• Teasing
• Unpopularity
• Prejudice
• Difficulty finding clothes
• Negative self-image
• Social withdrawal
• Increased risk of becoming an obese adult
• Increased risk of obesity-related illnesses (e.g., diabetes)
• Overestimation of the child's age by others, resulting in higher expectations that are a prelude to disappointment

In addition, treatment of obesity for this age group is difficult, in part because adolescence is such a difficult time.

Do I have a fat kid?

Adult measures of obesity that you have come to know and love, like the BMI and WHR, are not suitable for children and adolescents because they have different body composition. Instead, standard charts (available from your friendly local pediatrician) are used to evaluate optimum weight, height, and growth, and thereby identify overweight children. The tables on the next pages, derived from the National Health Center for Health Statistics, can help identify overweight children, in case obesity is not obvious from merely looking at them.

While there is no complete medical agree-ment on the definition of an overweight child, most pediatricians consider a child obese if he or she weighs more than 90 percent of children at the same height.

As shown in these tables, to determine a child's level of obesity, we measure the child's height in inches and identify the corresponding weight for that height. Weights greater than that of the 90th per-centile identify the overweight.

Note: Being overweight does not neces-sarily mean being obese, as the increased weight could be due to greater muscle or bone mass. You can confirm obesity, how-ever, by checking for increased skin-folds on the back of the arm, the shoulder blades, or the lower abdomen. Weight-management professionals use special calipers to accurately measure skin-folds.

Why kids become fat

Two factors are strongly associated with the development of childhood obesity. The chief factor is the amount of time spent watching television. Children who watch TV more than 2 hours per day have an increased risk of developing obesity, and this risk increases the more time they spend watching television.

Watching television is a very sedentary pastime that replaces physical activity. In this regard, working at computers or playing video games would create the same problems. While watching TV, children often eat high-fat foods. Also, television exposes children to fast-food commercials. Estimates say that the average child sees 10,000 food commercials per year, of which 95 percent are for fast food. Thus, spending time with computers and video games may be a healthier pursuit than television watching.

The other chief factor in the development of childhood obesity is the parents' weight. If one parent is obese, the child has a 40 percent chance of being obese. If both parents are obese, the risk increases to 80 percent. Other parental influences associated with increased childhood risk for obesity are inactivity, high socioeconomic class, and high level of education. Obesity also occurs more commonly in small families.

Prevention and treatment of childhood obesity

The first step in the treatment and prevention of any childhood problem is ensuring that parents and other family members provide a proper example to the child. You cannot expect a child to eat right or exercise if the parents are couch potatoes who survive on fast food. The single biggest component of treatment and prevention for this problem, therefore, rests in the home and with family ethics and habits. Parents should encourage healthy eating, increased physical activity, and decreased time in sedentary pursuits such as watching television, playing video games, and sitting at computers.

Specific treatment strategies

While good parenting examples are necessary for treatment, they may not be sufficient to treat the problem. An experienced pediatrician or family practitioner must be involved in treatment, and the whole family should be included in the management of the problem. Even more than with adults, the treatment of obese children must focus on behavior rather than weight. The overall strategy is to have children grow into their weight while changing their body composition—replacing fat with increased muscle mass and acquiring the bone density that comes naturally with age.

As a result, a child's weight loss per se should not be more than 1 pound per month. A weight-maintenance period of 1 to 2 years is also recommended for each 20 percent of weight loss. A behavior modification specialist should train the family and the child to change behavior along the lines suggested in the Lifestyle chapter of this book, including changes that involve self-management, motivation, craving control, and rewards.

It is important to recognize that children will have times of increased appetite dictated by growth spurts and other developmental needs. An emphasis on healthy

Obesity in Younger Children

Weight for Height

Boys

Height (inches)	Normal weight (lbs.) 50th percentile (average)	120% x normal weight (lbs.) 90th percentile (overweight)
34	28	33
36	30	35
38	32	38
40	35	42
42	39	47
44	43	52
46	46	56
48	51	61
50	55	67
52	61	74

Girls

Height (inches)	Normal weight (lbs.) 50th percentile (average)	120% x normal weight (lbs.) 90th percentile (overweight)
34	26	31
36	29	35
38	31	38
40	34	41
42	39	46
44	41	49
46	46	55
48	49	59
50	55	66
52	62	74
54	69	83

Obesity in Older Children

Weight for Height

Boys

Height (inches)	Normal weight (lbs.) 50th percentile (average)	120% x normal weight (lbs.) 90th percentile (overweight)
54	66	82
56	76	91
58	85	102
60	93	111
62	101	129
64	111	133
66	121	145
68	135	162
70	151	182

Girls

Height (inches)	Normal weight (lbs.) 50th percentile (average)	120% x normal weight (lbs.) 90th percentile (overweight)
56	77	92
57	81	97
58	85	102
59	88	107
60	94	113
61	97	117
62	102	122
63	110	132
64	119	144

eating rather than reduced eating is thus even more crucial for the child than it is for the adult. At this age, food volume is less important than food quality.

Physical activity is a crucial aspect of any weight-loss program, and this is no less the case for children. Children should be encouraged to stay active. While many overweight children may not like conventional team sports, they can still enjoy walking, swimming, or biking. Formal exercise classes might be useful but would require the supervision of a qualified exercise instructor familiar with the needs of this age group. Informal activities like community "fun runs" and walks where everyone gets a ribbon are particularly good for this age group.

Weight training can only minimally increase muscle strength or mass in children. Lifting too much weight can actually injure young bones. Adolescents who want to start weight training should learn proper technique from a qualified instructor and stay with a low-weight, high-repetition routine until their bodies mature.

Informal exercise and activity is still the preferred route for children. And don't forget—you must set a good example, too!

Anti-obesity drugs and surgical methods are definitely not recommended for this group. Both drugs and surgical interventions would hinder normal physical and psychological development.

The elderly

As we age, muscle mass decreases, slowing metabolism; we require fewer calories. This trend, along with the tendency of many people to become less active as they age, obviously creates a danger of weight gain as we get older. And excess weight compounds the natural problems of aging. Conversely, being slim reduces some of the problems inherent in aging. Eating a healthy diet and being active are associated with a much better quality of life, including better mobility and improved cognitive skills.

Special Considerations for the Elderly

With aging, some individuals experience low levels of calcium in their bones, resulting in bone thinning (osteoporosis), which may be aggravated by weight loss. Exercise should be supervised to avoid bone fractures.

Medical conditions common in the elderly, like lazy thyroid or depression, require professional consultation and treatment.

Restricting calories while taking water pills (diuretics) could cause a drop in blood pressure, so fluid intake should be increased.

The number of taste buds decreases with age, and this particularly affects salty and sweet tastes. As a result, older people may be more likely to overconsume salty or sweet foods, leading to increased calorie intake.

Food and the elderly

The elderly have special dietary requirements:

- Older persons should not reduce their intake below 1,200 calories a day.
- To preserve muscle mass, they should eat at least 70 grams of protein each day.
- Complex carbohydrates should account for about 60 percent of total intake.
- Calcium intake, required to keep bones healthy, should be between 1,200 and 1,500 milligrams per day.
- Vitamin supplements are often necessary to avoid deficiencies.

Exercise and the elderly

It is absolutely essential that anyone embarking on an exercise program in this age group consult with a physician first to determine an appropriate activity level. An exercise tolerance test or other cardio-vascular stress test is sometimes needed.

Any activity, as long as it is safe, can be beneficial, no matter how limited it may appear.

Resistance exercises (e.g., using hand-held weights, performing aqua exercises) are extremely valuable for preserving muscle mass and maintaining bone density. These are almost essential, especially for older women, who are at increased risk of osteoporosis.

Overall muscle strength decreases slightly with age. Even at the age of sixty, however, maximum muscle strength has only declined 10 to 20 percent from the maxi-mum strength at age thirty. People in their seventies and eighties can take up a weight-resistance program and gain strength along with some increase in muscle size.

Stretching and flexibility exercises are valuable for preserving muscle tone, improving circulation, and maintaining maximum mobility.

Walking, no matter how slowly, is an excellent basic exercise for mobility and for reducing the risk of cardiovascular and other diseases. It is important to note that older people do not have to exercise quite as hard to get a training effect. As a result, older individuals should start at very low heart levels (under 100 beats per minute) and increase progressively. (The target rate should be adjusted for those taking medication that reduces the pulse.)

Exercise is the single biggest behavior that can improve the life of the elderly. With better mobility and overall health, there is less likelihood of social withdrawal and thus depression. The trainability of an older individual is roughly equivalent to that of a young adult. When properly and safely done, exercise can improve the older person's mental and physical abilities as well as his or her spirit.

Pregnant and lactating women

Pregnancy is, of course, associated with weight gain. It is one of the few times when weight gain is necessary for normal, healthy development. While some weight gain is essential during pregnancy, too much weight gained during this time can lead to serious obesity problems. In fact, an impor-tant part of the obstetrician's prenatal examination is the calculation of BMI.

The recommendations for weight gain during pregnancy vary, depending on how overweight the mother is to begin with.

For a woman with a pre-pregnancy BMI of 26 to 29, the optimal maternal weight gain during pregnancy is 0.7 pounds per week. This allows a total gain of 28 pounds during a full-term pregnancy.

For a woman whose pre-pregnancy BMI is 30 or more, a weight gain of 0.5 pounds per week is recommended. This allows for a total weight gain of 20 pounds during a full-term pregnancy.

Pregnancy itself causes some weight gain, but some mothers tend to see pregnancy as a reason to lift their normal dietary restraint and indulge in "eating for two."

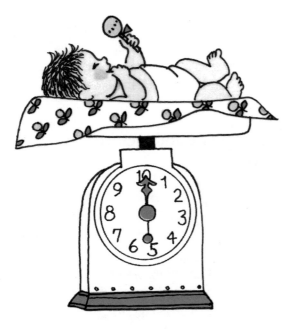

Pregnancy is often the beginning of significant weight gain. Gaining excessive weight during pregnancy increases the risk of postnatal obesity. Research shows that women who gain 35 pounds during pregnancy on average remain approximately 11 pounds above their pre-pregnancy weight 6 to 12 months after delivery.

Obese Mothers Are More Likely to...

- Need labor induction or Caesarean delivery
- Develop mild or severe toxemias of pregnancy (preeclampsia, eclampsia)
- Become diabetic or hypertensive
- Deliver larger babies

The goal of the overweight mother-to-be should be to avoid gaining more weight than is necessary beyond the optimal 20 to 28 pounds. The pregnant woman should eat a healthy diet with adequate, not excessive, calories. This is typically achieved by eating an extra 600 calories a day, assuming that the pre-pregnancy diet was a healthy one. In addition, the pregnant woman should add 30 grams of protein to her diet.

Pregnancy is not a time to try to lose weight. It is a time to eat healthily and exercise sensibly. If a woman is concerned about her weight, she should limit her weight-reduction efforts to before pregnancy or after breast-feeding.

Many doctors now give the okay to exercise during pregnancy. A woman who was exercising regularly before pregnancy can continue to do so moderately at least three times a week for 15 minutes, unless there is a medical reason not to.

A woman who was a pre-pregnancy exerciser will need to modify the intensity and type of exercise as her body changes. Swimming is an excellent exercise during pregnancy because it can be done so much more comfortably than many other activities.

A pregnant woman who is not used to exercising should not engage in any activity more demanding than walking.

The Pregnant Woman Should...

- Avoid exercising in hot, humid weather.

- Ensure that her body temperature stays below 101 degrees.

- Drink lots of water.

- Keep her heart rate no higher than 70 percent of peak capacity and in any event, no higher than 140 beats per minute.

- Avoid jarring movements and overextension of joints.

- Avoid exercises that involve lying on her back (after the fourth month of pregnancy); these can impede blood flow to the baby.

- Listen to her body and stop exercising if there is any pain, dizziness, bleeding, or shortness of breath.

People with hormonal abnormalities

Obesity in women is sometimes associated with abnormal levels of male and female sex hormones. This can result in:
- Menstrual irregularities
- Hirsutism—hair growth in male patterns (i.e., on the face and chest)
- Formation of small ovarian cysts, a condition called polycystic ovary
- Reduced fertility

Weight loss can alleviate these conditions.

Obesity in men is also sometimes associated with abnormal levels of both male and female hormones. This can result in:
- Diminished sperm count and reduced fertility
- Diminished sexual desire

These conditions, too, can be improved by weight reduction.

Menopausal women

Menopause is the time of life when the ovaries stop producing female hormones. This decline is often accompanied by episodes of flushing, irritability, low self-esteem, and occasional fatigue or depression.

During menopause, muscle mass begins to decrease, and as a result, metabolism slows and caloric requirements are reduced. This often leads to weight gain, especially around the waist. It is also a time when women begin to show symptoms of common obesity complications such as diabetes, hypertension, and heart disease.

Menopause is an important milestone in a woman's life, with psychological and physical implications. The support of family and friends is valuable. So is the skill and support of a physician. The physician plays an important role at this stage by providing periodic checkups for early diagnosis and treatment of obesity-related conditions, and by determining the wisdom of hormone replacement therapy and following up if therapy is indicated.

The nutritional recommendations made throughout this book apply just as well at this stage of life. There are two essential considerations, however:

- Daily calcium intake should total 1,000 to 1,500 milligrams a day.
- Resistance workouts are especially important, because they will preserve muscle mass.

People with limited mobility

People who have limited mobility and/or are confined to wheelchairs are at special risk for developing obesity because of their severely reduced opportunities for calorie-burning activity. In addition, their muscle mass is decreased, thus reducing metabolism even further. As a result, the caloric requirements of this group are low, and caloric intake has to be adjusted accordingly. The psychological effects of confinement can lead to depression and poor motivation. And let's not forget the effect of the physical injury or illness that led to the confinement in the first place.

Obviously, the involvement of a physician is important. A dietitian will help by recommending a suitably low-fat diet that will meet nutritional needs.

Exercise is the most important component for this group. A physical rehabilitation specialist can provide excellent advice and instruction on exercises that can be done when confined.

Below are descriptions of typical exercises that can be accomplished by a person with upper body mobility who is confined to a wheelchair.

Elbow-arm extensions for neck rotation and shoulder/elbow mobility: Place right hand on chair seat, left hand across right shoulder. Turn head to right. Extend left arm beyond left shoulder while turning head to left. Return to starting position. Repeat ten times with each arm.

Elbow-shoulder stretches to stretch and strengthen chest and shoulder muscles: Clasp hands behind neck with elbows together in front of chin. Keeping elbows at chin level, bring them out and back as far as possible. Repeat up to ten times.

Hand-trunk stretches to stretch lower back and increase shoulder mobility: With feet on footrests, hold right armrest or back of seat with right hand. Sit up, then bend forward from the waist, reaching down with left hand as far as you can. Hold for about six counts, without bouncing, then sit up again. Repeat five times with each arm.

Wheelchair push-ups for triceps, abdominal, and forearm muscles: Place hands on wheel rims or armrests. Straighten elbows to lift body out of chair. Lower body to count of four. Repeat up to ten times. To strengthen abdominals, lift body out of chair, swing hips to the right and then to the left before sitting back down.

Depressed people

As noted in the Lifestyle chapter, there are many forms of depression. Regardless of whether a person's depression has a biological basis or is a natural reaction to life circumstances, energy is drained. Without energy, outlook becomes far more negative, self-esteem sinks, and feelings of despair arise.

Severe forms of depression tend to reduce appetite, leading to weight loss. In the more common types of depression, however, eating tends to increase, because:
• The body seeks food to get more energy.
• The depressed person tries to fill the emotional emptiness with physical fullness.
• During periods of withdrawal and isolation, eating is a stimulating behavior.
• Food blocks out depressed feelings.

Depression can be successfully treated with a combination of antidepressant drugs and counseling. Although weight loss increases self-esteem, the chances of successfully embarking on a weight-loss program while depressed are poor. It is crucial, then, that treatment for depression precede any weight-loss attempt. Nonetheless, several measures that fight depression will also help a weight problem. Factors to consider include:

Exercise: The best way to increase energy is to exercise. Given that depression is an energy problem, it is clear that exercising is an important part of a fight against depression. In fact, exercise is now a standard treatment for depression. Of course, motivating oneself to exercise, or to do anything, when depressed is the real trick. Others can help the depressed person get going. Personal trainers and friends who won't take no for an answer are the most helpful in this situation.

Low sugar and caffeine intake: Both of these substances give a quick fix of energy in the short term but deplete energy thereafter. Clearly, it's not desirable to deplete energy if you have an energy problem to begin with.

Medications: Some antidepressant medications reduce cravings and appetite, others increase them, and still others have little effect at all. Moreover, people have vast individual differences in their reactions to these drugs. Anyone subject to depression should consult a physician about this aspect of medication before accepting a prescription for any drugs.

Counseling: Counseling can help the depressed person understand more about the relationship between moods, thoughts, and behavior, including eating behavior. Cognitive therapy, the most valuable therapeutic technique for depression, will also help control eating and manage weight.

Obesity-related diseases

Diabetes mellitus

Diabetes mellitus is a condition in which the body can no longer satisfactorily manage glucose use and storage. If not treated properly, diabetes can lead to serious complications, including blindness, kidney failure, heart disease, foot ulcers, and the need for limb amputations.

In non-diabetic individuals, blood sugar (glucose) levels after an overnight fast fall within the range of 80 to 110 milligrams percent. The overnight fast blood sugar measure is known as the *basal level*. After a meal, blood sugar increases before returning to its basal level within 3 hours. In diabetic individuals, basal blood glucose is high, rises higher after eating, and takes longer than normal to return to basal levels.

Glucose levels are controlled by the hormone insulin, which is produced by the pancreas. Insulin helps drive the glucose out of the blood for use and subsequent storage. After eating, blood sugar levels rise, signaling to the pancreas to produce insulin. Insulin then activates muscles to utilize glucose for energy. Liver and fat cells store what cannot be used for energy.

There are two forms of diabetes: adult-onset and juvenile-onset.

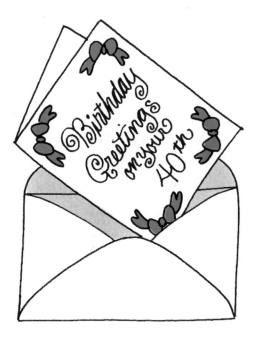

Adult-onset diabetes

Adult-onset diabetes usually begins after age forty. This is the type of diabetes that occurs with obesity. In fact, 80 percent of those suffering from adult-onset diabetes are obese.

This type of diabetes is also called type 2 diabetes or non-insulin-dependent diabetes mellitus (NIDDM). It is called NIDDM because the treatment regimen rarely requires insulin.

Adult-onset diabetes results from a reduction in the ability of the body, and especially the muscles, to respond to insulin. This state is called *insulin resistance*.

Obese individuals develop insulin resistance long before the symptoms of diabetes surface. Early stages of the condition create mild and vague symptoms of fatigue, making early diagnosis unlikely. The disease begins with the development of insulin resistance. The pancreas produces more of the hormone to compensate for this resistance. Eventually, as insulin resistance gets worse, the pancreas cannot keep up with the increased insulin demand, and blood sugar rises. As this process continues, the pancreas becomes exhausted and cannot recognize the body's need to get rid of sugar. As a result, insulin production decreases, and blood sugar levels continue to rise to the point where the basal level is much higher than normal.

Risk factors for adult-onset diabetes include:

• *Strong family history of diabetes.*
  Diabetes is mediated by genes that influence both the production of insulin by the pancreas and the body's responsiveness to insulin.

- *Race.* People of certain races are more disposed to developing diabetes with obesity, including American Indians, Hispanics, and African Americans/Canadians.

- *Pregnancy-related factors.* Abnormal increases in blood glucose during pregnancy and the delivery of a baby weighing over 9 pounds are indicators of subsequent diabetic problems.

- *Obesity.* Being obese increases the risk threefold. Having excess fat around the waist further increases the risk by another three times.

Juvenile-onset diabetes

Can you guess why juvenile-onset diabetes is thus named? Yes, you're right! This condition typically begins at a young age, often in late adolescence. It is fundamentally different from adult-onset diabetes in that it results primarily from the destruction of the cells in the pancreas that produce insulin. As a result, people with this condition need to provide insulin for their bodies, and so this form of the condition is called insulin-dependent diabetes mellitus (IDDM). This condition is also called type 1 diabetes and is uncommon among the obese.

Diagnosis and treatment of adult-onset diabetes

The diagnosis of diabetes is easily made by measuring blood glucose either randomly or after a fast. "Borderline" or "impaired glucose tolerance" is the diagnosis when fasting glucose is 110 to 126 mg percent or random glucose is 126 to 200 mg percent. "Overt" diabetes is considered present when fasting glucose is greater than 126 mg percent or random glucose is greater than 200 mg percent.

If there is any doubt about the diagnosis, a standard medical test, the oral glucose tolerance test (OGTT), is conducted. The patient drinks a beverage containing 75 grams of glucose. Blood samples are taken after 30 minutes, 1 hour, $1^{1}/2$ hours, and 2 hours. Diabetes is present if the blood glucose level is over 200 mg percent 2 hours after drinking the beverage. Values above 140 during the period of the test identify individuals who either have borderline diabetes or are likely to develop diabetes in the future.

Treatment consists of a weight-reduction and exercise program such as the one outlined in this guide. Weight losses of 5 to 10 percent of body weight substantially improve the opportunity for successful treatment.

If the patient does not lose weight, the physician can prescribe one of several oral medications that treat NIDDM (non-insulin-dependent diabetes mellitus). Insulin is used only as a last resort.

Special considerations

One of the central problems with diabetes is, of course, high blood sugar levels. It is important, therefore, to do what's necessary to keep blood sugar levels as low as possible, including:
- Avoiding sugary foods
- Eating small meals. This prevents blood-sugar levels from getting too high.
- Not skipping meals. Skipping meals increases hunger, so the person is more likely to make unhealthy choices as well as to eat a greater volume of food. The bigger the meal, the higher the blood sugar.
- Minimizing stress. Blood sugar levels rise with stress.

Some of the medications used to treat diabetes, as well as insulin itself, interfere with weight reduction. It is important, therefore, to lose as much weight as possible before embarking on these drugs.

Regular checkups with a physician are important. The physician will monitor progress and check for associated conditions like heart disease and hypertension.

Hypertension

Hypertension is often called the "silent disease" because its symptoms often are not noticeable to the patient. The illness is defined as a continuously elevated blood pressure. The heart is forced to work harder, and this can lead to heart disease and eventual heart failure. Also, many other organs, including the brain and kidneys, can be severely affected by hypertension.

Hypertension affects millions of people. The prevalence of hypertension in obese individuals is 25 to 50 percent, three times higher than in non-obese people.

Why is hypertension more common in obese people?

As noted in the section on diabetes, obese people increase their levels of insulin in response to insulin resistance. The high blood insulin level can cause the kidneys to retain salt and water, which increases blood volume, thus increasing the pressure that the blood exerts on veins and arteries.

Other factors that increase the risk of developing hypertension include:
• A strong family history of hypertension
• Excess fat around the waist
  (apple-shaped obesity)
• Diabetes mellitus

• High blood cholesterol
• Cigarette smoking
• Excessive alcohol use

Diagnosis and treatment of hypertension

Hypertension is simply diagnosed by taking blood pressure on several occasions. Although you may have had your blood pressure measured many times, you almost certainly can't spell the name of the instrument used to measure it—the sphygmomanometer. This device generates two numbers, usually expressed as a fraction. *Systolic pressure* is measured when the heart is contracting; this generates the top number of the fraction. *Diastolic pressure* is measured when the heart is relaxing; this generates the number at the bottom of the fraction.

Hypertension is present when repeated measures show:
• Systolic pressure greater than 140 mmHg
• Diastolic pressure greater than 90 mmHg

The criteria for someone with diabetes are slightly less: systolic pressure of 135 mmHg and diastolic pressure of 85 mmHg.

The treatment of hypertension, of course, involves a healthy diet and a sensible exercise regimen. Both weight reduction and exercise have been shown to separately reduce hypertension significantly and can often reduce or eliminate the need for drug treatments. And speaking of drug treatments, several available medications reduce hypertension, but some of these worsen insulin resistance, so the physician should do a thorough screening before making the appropriate choice.

The most important dietary consideration for hypertensives, apart from a low-fat diet, is the restriction of salt. Salt increases blood volume still further, exacerbating hypertension. Eliminating salt from the diet is a critical component in the treatment regime.

Heart disease and stroke

Fats are carried around the blood in particles known as lipoproteins. Lipoproteins can penetrate arterial walls and deposit their fat. These fat deposits cause repeated cycles of irritation and healing which eventually lead to thinning and then hardening of the arteries, a disease called atherosclerosis.

Thinned blood vessels can rupture easily, especially if blood pressure is high. This may cause bleeding in such vital organs as the brain, leading to stroke or death. Hardening of blood vessels can also lead to blood clots that can block blood supply to the heart (causing heart attack) or the brain (causing stroke).

Am I at risk?

The risk factors associated with high blood fats and coronary disease are:

- *Age*. Men over forty-five and women over fifty-five are at risk.

- *Family history*. Those with a strong family history of high blood fats and/or coronary artery disease have increased risk.

- *Smoking*. Cigarette smokers have an elevated risk.

- *Inactivity*. A sedentary lifestyle is associated with increased risk.

- *Obesity-related diseases*. Diabetes and hypertension sufferers are more at risk. In fact, diabetes counts as two risk factors.

- *Weight*. Women who have a BMI greater than 30 are twice as likely to have these problems than women whose BMI is between 25 and 30.

- *Fat distribution*. Apple shapes are more at risk for coronary heart disease.

- *Cholesterol ratios*. Cholesterol consists of high-density lipoproteins (HDL), known as "good cholesterol," and low density lipoproteins (LDL), known as "bad" cholesterol. The greater the proportion of HDL in the blood, the better. Ratios are determined by the formula:

Total cholesterol divided by HDL

For example, if your total cholesterol was 200 and your HDL was 50, your ratio would be:

200 divided by 50 = 4

If, however, your total cholesterol was 200 and your HDL was 20, your ratio would be:

200 divided by 20 = 10

Clearly, there is a vastly different clinical picture between these two examples. A ratio of 4 is roughly normal, but a ratio of 10 is grossly abnormal and would indicate significantly higher risk.

Diagnosis and treatment

The diagnosis of undesirable fat levels in the blood is made by testing the blood after an overnight fast.

The criteria for undesirable blood fat levels are:

- Total cholesterol greater than 200 mg percent

- LDL cholesterol:
  —Greater than 100 mg percent if the person already has heart disease
  —Greater than 130 mg percent if the person has two or more risk factors for heart disease
  —Greater than 160 mg percent if the person has no other risk factors for heart disease

- HDL cholesterol less than 35 mg percent

- Triglycerides greater than 250 mg percent

Weight reduction is the cornerstone of treatment for this condition. In particular, the reduction of saturated fat and cholesterol intake is a critical goal, often set in collaboration with a dietary counselor.

Exercise is also a critical treatment component, because exercise has been shown to increase the proportion of HDL, the "good" cholesterol.

Through a low-fat diet and a sensible exercise program, overall blood fat levels can be reduced, often significantly, and sometimes very quickly. If the person does not embark on a sensible weight-loss program or does so but is unsuccessful in reducing blood fat levels, medications can help control the condition.

Because smoking is an associated risk factor, smoking cessation is also an essential treatment component.

The physician's role in the treatment process involves:
- Screening and treatment of associated conditions such as NIDDM and hypertension
- Screening and testing to determine suitable levels of exercise
- Prescription and monitoring of medications
- Smoking cessation advice and support

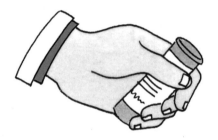

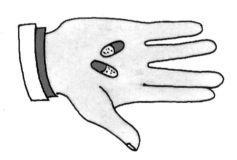

Gall bladder disease

Your gall bladder is a sac, situated just above your stomach, which stores bile produced by the liver. Your liver releases bile into the gut to aid the digestive process. Normally, cholesterol is dissolved in the bile and removed from the body, but when this does not happen efficiently, gallstones form. These gallstones irritate the bile duct, the canal leading from the gall bladder to the gut, and gall bladder disease results from this repeated irritation.

Obesity is associated with increased cholesterol levels in the bile. Women with a BMI greater than 30 have at least twice the risk of developing gallstones as women with a BMI below 25. Gall bladder disease is particularly common in obese middle-aged women who have had multiple pregnancies.

Although weight reduction is necessary for people who are obese, *rapid weight loss can actually cause gallstone formation*. As a result, people with a history of gall bladder disease should be warned about the dangers of rapid weight reduction. Gallstones and gall bladder disease should be treated before weight loss is attempted.

Osteoarthritis and gout

Osteoarthritis and gout are diseases of the joints. Osteoarthritis is the most common form of arthritis. It occurs when there is excessive wear of joint cartilage and its smooth lubricated coverings. Obviously, carrying excessive weight can stress joints, and you will not be surprised to learn that osteoarthritis is more common in obese than non-obese people. Poor posture, occupational stresses, and other factors can also increase the risk of osteoarthritis. Weight loss can reduce the stress on joints and can also reduce the amount of medication required to treat this condition.

Gout is another joint disease. When digested, certain foods such as liver, kidneys, and sweetbreads break down into a product called uric acid. Excess uric acid creates gout, a painful condition that affects mostly men but also affects postmenopausal women. People suffering from gout should drink a lot of fluids during any weight-reduction program. The increase in water volume excreted will help to remove uric acid from the blood, decreasing the risk of it being deposited in the joints. This practice will also help to prevent its deposition in the kidneys and therefore decrease the chances of forming some types of kidney stones.

Cancer

Cancer results from changes in the growth of cells, which grow abnormally and rapidly, overwhelming the normal cells in their part of the body. The genes that typically limit cell growth have been implicated in the development of these tumors. Exactly how the normal genetic process is disturbed is not clear, but certain agents are known to have a carcinogenic effect. These agents include irritants like tar in cigarette smoke; radiation, such as ultraviolet or X-rays; and certain viruses. The growth of some types of cancer is associated with consumption of particular nutrients (e.g., fat) or abnormal levels of hormones (e.g., estrogen or testosterone).

Cancer can occur in any part of the body. Types of cancer specifically related to obesity are cancer of the breast and womb in women, and cancer of the prostate and colon in men.

The reason for the increased cancer risk in obesity is unclear. It might be associated with a high intake of fat or some other nutrient, or it might be associated with obesity itself. Cancer of the reproductive organs in women might result from increased estrogen production by fat tissue. Obese women have higher levels of estrogen in their blood. If their obesity occurred in childhood, these women would have reached puberty sooner. And obese women become menopausal later in life than non-obese women. So it is conceivable that obese women have a higher and longer exposure to estrogen, and this may increase their cancer risk.

Breast cancer is not only related to estrogen levels but also to total body fat and body composition. Apple shapes are more prone to breast cancer than others.

Prevention
Prevention and early detection are the best ways of handling cancer. The six keys to doing this are as follows:
• Undergo regular, routine screening.
• Avoid contact with known carcinogens, such as cigarette smoke or organic solvents.
• Avoid excessive exposure to all forms of radiation, including strong sunlight.
• Reduce weight and excess body fat.
• Eat a low-fat diet rich in fruits and vegetables.
• Adopt a sensible exercise regimen as outlined in this guide.

Bulimia
Bulimia is an eating disorder associated with the development of obesity. In the Lifestyle chapter, we discussed the dynamics and treatment of binge eating disorder. Bulimia involves many of the same dynamics, and its treatment is similar to that outlined for binge eating.

The main difference between bulimia and binge eating disorder is that bulimics attempt to offset the effects of their bingeing through compensatory behaviors such as self-induced vomiting, diuretic abuse, excessive laxative use, and compulsive exercise. In addition, bulimics tend to have a greater risk for alcohol and drug use, self-injurious behavior, depression, and compulsive behavior, including compulsive sexual problems.

Besides these behavioral and psychological difficulties, bulimics often have physical problems that result from their compensatory behaviors, including:
• *Gastric reflux.* With repeated purging, the body begins to regurgitate food automatically.
• *Swollen salivary glands.* Repeated vomiting enlarges the salivary glands, resulting in swelling under the jawline.
• *Stained teeth.* Repeated vomiting erodes tooth enamel.
• *Finger clubbing.* Swelling results when the fingers used to induce vomiting come into contact with the acid that accompanies regurgitation.

How does bulimia start?
Like most eating disorders, bulimia begins in adolescence. There are two high-risk periods in the development of bulimia. The first occurs in early adolescence at the beginning of puberty, a time of great

physical change. The second occurs a little later on, typically at the later stages of high school or early in college, a time of great social change.

Bulimia obviously accompanies concern with weight. Preoccupation with weight can occur because of pressure from friends and family but also from the pursuit of activities where thinness is an advantage. To that end, ballet dancing, modeling, and gymnastics are all high-risk behaviors where being thin or even underweight may be encouraged by coaches and other interested parties. The compensatory behaviors of bulimia are often learned from "friends."

Diagnosis and treatment of bulimia

Typical bulimic behaviors that help identify the condition are:
- Recurrent episodes of binge eating—typically a large amount of food in a discrete time period, often less than two hours
- Bingeing on high-calorie food
- Bingeing in private
- Bingeing that continues until the person experiences pain, falls asleep, runs out of food, is interrupted, or vomits
- Repeated attempts to lose weight by severely restrictive diets
- Self-induced vomiting; excessive laxative or diuretic use
- Rapid and frequent weight fluctuations greater than 10 pounds as a result of alternating binges and fasts
- Awareness that eating pattern is abnormal
- Feelings of shame, guilt, and worthlessness following a binge

Overweight bulimics require special treatment. It is not advisable for a bulimic to embark on a weight-loss program without consideration and treatment of several key issues, particularly the chaos and impulsiveness that characterize this condition.

Treatment of bulimia, like the treatment of binge eating disorder mentioned earlier, involves counseling to address the extreme perfectionism and all-or-nothing thinking that is typical of someone with this condition. In addition, counseling needs to address the underlying emotions that are being avoided through the use of impulsive behaviors.

Depression is common in bulimics. Antidepressant medications and cognitive therapy help alleviate bulimic symptoms. Also, estimates are that about 30 percent of bulimics have suffered childhood trauma, often of a sexual nature. Therapy needs to address and resolve these issues.

Behavioral retraining is critical for successful treatment. Initially, retraining is aimed at eliminating self-injurious behavior, like self-induced vomiting, and establishing sensible exercise and eating patterns. Identifying and managing high-risk situations is critical, as is therapy for distorted body image—because bulimics often have ambivalent feelings about their bodies. Individual and group therapy can address this problem. Family therapy is also useful in addressing the control and power issues that frequently accompany bulimia.

All of these treatment components can make an effective therapeutic package. Short-term reduction of bingeing can frequently be achieved, and the modification of impulsive behaviors, as well as treatment for underlying depression, can have substantial long-term effects.

A quiz on strategies for special needs

1) What is a normal basal blood sugar level?
2) What is the daily protein requirement of an elderly person?
3) Overt diabetes is diagnosed when fasting glucose is greater than what level?
4) What is the range of acceptable weight gain during pregnancy?
5) Which cancers are specifically related to obesity in women?

Answers:
1) 80 to 110 mg percent
2) 70 grams
3) 126 mg percent
4) 20 to 28 pounds
5) Cancer of the breast and womb

28-DAY GUIDE

INTRODUCTION

Previous pages of this guidebook have provided the information, skills, and advice you need to lose weight and maintain a healthy weight. This section puts it all together in a powerful 28-day program that will reinforce the important information you have already learned and provide training in critical motivational and behavioral skills. A menu plan, nutritional tips, and a fitness guide are also included, all of which make getting started on a weight-loss program as easy as you can say TOPS. The program is great if you are trying to get started or restarted, or if you just want a change in your routine. It is designed for those who want to lose weight as well as those who want to maintain their losses.

We strongly recommend that you read the entire guide before you begin this program. The guide provides detailed information and advice.

The elements of this 28-day program are:

- A daily "affirmation": A catchy, meaningful phrase to remind you of important goals. Repeat your affirmation frequently during the day.
- A key fact to "remember": This will remind you of important medical, nutritional, fitness, and lifestyle information.
- Some "do" assignments which will help you monitor energy intake and expenditure.

- A blank Daily Journal page for "recording" your progress, observations, and triumphs. (Photocopy this page for daily use.)
- A "menu for the day" providing three meals and a snack geared to three intake levels—1,200; 1,500; and 1,800 calories.

IMPORTANT

We have taken extra steps to use some of the new, very lean meat exchanges. Their low calorie level (35 calories per ounce) allow the menus to be more flexible with the meat exchanges—occasionally exceeding the meat exchange limit as listed in the Sample Exchange Lists on page 40. When you apply this to your own menus, keep total meat calories in mind. Individuals on the 1,200- or 1,500-calorie exchange plan should not exceed 300 total meat calories; those on the 1,800-calorie plan should limit themselves to 400 total meat calories.

We recommend that you repeat the 28-day program at least three times. The steps should become part of your daily routine. If you begin the program and then stop for more than a few days, we suggest you restart the program from Day 1.

Good luck!

THE DAILY JOURNAL

Keeping a daily journal is an important way to monitor your behavior and assess your progress. Use the format below and/or the TOPS exchange recorder to keep track of your own program or the 28-day program provided with this guide. Photocopy this page or order your reusable exchange recorder (item M-7) through your chapter (form L-15).

Date: _____ **Daily intake goals:** _____ **Daily exercise expenditure goal:** _____

Food Consumed:

Meal	Food/amount	Fat gm	Cals.
Breakfast			
Lunch			
Dinner			
Snacks			
TOTAL			

Comments:

Exercise Done:

Exercise	Time	Time spent	Calories burned
Other activities			
TOTAL			

Comments:

DAY 1

Affirmation: Taking control of my weight and my health is my number one priority.

Remember: Make an appointment with my physician.

Do: DIET: Purchase the foods I will need for this week's menu.
EXERCISE: Do warm-up and cool-down routines.
LIFESTYLE: Practice deep-breathing exercises for 5 minutes.

Record: Food intake, calories, and fat grams
Calories burned

MENU FOR THE DAY

	Breakfast	Lunch	Dinner	Snack
1,200 calorie menu	1 slice diet bread 2 tsp. sugar-free jelly 1 1/4 cups strawberries 1 cup plain yogurt, nonfat, sugar-free Free foods	3 oz. water-packed tuna on 2 slices diet whole-wheat bread with Lettuce leaves 1 tsp. margarine 1 cup tomato soup 1 small apple 1 cup nonfat milk	4 oz. poached haddock 1 cup steamed carrots 1/2 medium baked potato 2 tsp. margarine 1 slice plain angel food cake* Free foods	1 fruit exchange Free foods
1,500 calorie menu **ADD to 1,200 menu:**		1 starch/bread exchange 2 vegetable exchanges		1 fruit exchange
1,800 calorie menu **ADD to 1,500 menu:**			1 meat exchange 2 fat exchanges	1 fruit exchange

* Purchase whole angel food cake. Cut into 12 slices. Wrap and freeze individual slices.
Note portion sizes of free foods. Portions beyond these sizes are NOT free!

137

DAY 2

Affirmation: If I am wise, I will exercise.
Remember: Measure my BMI.

Do: DIET: Make a list of foods I enjoy from each of the six exchange groups.
            This will be my resource for developing my own menus later.
            EXERCISE: Do warm-up and cool-down routines. Assess my flexibility level.
            LIFESTYLE: Spend 10 minutes practicing craving-control imagery.

Record: Food intake, calories, and fat grams
            Calories burned

MENU FOR THE DAY

	Breakfast	Lunch	Dinner	Snack
1,200 calorie menu	2/3 cup oatmeal 2 Tbsp. raisins 1 cup nonfat milk Free foods	1 oz. sandwich meat (1 g fat or less) on 2 slices diet bread with Lettuce leaves 1 tsp. margarine 1 cup chicken noodle soup 1 cup peaches in own juice Free foods	4-oz. skinless chicken breast (baked) 1/2 cup mashed potatoes mixed with 1/2 cup mashed carrots 1/2 cup steamed broccoli 2 tsp. margarine Free foods	1 starch/bread exchange 1 milk exchange Free foods
1,500 calorie menu **ADD to 1,200 menu:**		1 vegetable exchange	1 starch/bread exchange	1 fruit exchange 1 vegetable exchange
1,800 calorie menu **ADD to 1,500 menu:**		1 starch/bread exchange 1 vegetable exchange	1 meat exchange 2 fat exchanges	1 fruit exchange

Note portion sizes of free foods. Portions beyond these sizes are NOT free!

DAY 3

Affirmation: A healthy snack can keep me on track.

Remember: Visualize my serving size.

Do: DIET: Consult my list of favorite foods from each exchange. Write the exact size of a single serving next to each item.
This will be my resource for developing my own menus later.
EXERCISE: Do warm-up and cool-down routines. Assess my strength level.
LIFESTYLE: Spend 15 minutes practicing the meditation exercises.

Record: Food intake, calories, and fat grams
Calories burned

MENU FOR THE DAY

	Breakfast	Lunch	Dinner	Snack
1,200 calorie menu	3/4 cup Total cereal 1 small banana 1/2 cup nonfat milk Free foods	1/2 cup 4-5% fat cottage cheese 1 cup mixed fruit 4 Ry Krisp crackers 1 cup raw carrots & celery 1/4 cup salsa 1/2 cup nonfat milk Free foods	3 oz. lean roast beef* 1 cup mashed potatoes 1/2 tsp. margarine 1/3 cup peas Sugar-free gelatin Free foods	1 milk exchange Free foods
1,500 calorie menu **ADD to 1,200 menu:**		1 starch/bread exchange 1 vegetable exchange	1 vegetable exchange	1 fruit exchange
1,800 calorie menu **ADD to 1,500 menu:**			1 meat exchange 1 fat exchange	1 fruit exchange 1 fat exchange

* Cook entire roast. Slice in 1-oz. servings so I can choose portion sizes for now and later. Freeze what I do not need today.
Note portion sizes of free foods. Portions beyond these sizes are NOT free!

139

DAY 4

Affirmation: I choose reachable targets; they make the best goals.

Remember: Have my physician work with me to help establish my weight-loss goal.

Do: DIET: Review the favorite foods I have listed for each exchange group.
Replace two high-fat or high-sugar foods with fat-free or sugar-free substitutes.
EXERCISE: Do warm-up and cool-down routines. Assess my aerobic fitness level.
LIFESTYLE: Spend 15 minutes implementing the anger-control imagery.

Record: Food intake, calories, and fat grams
Calories burned

MENU FOR THE DAY

	Breakfast	Lunch	Dinner	Snack
1,200 calorie menu	2 slices raisin toast 1 tsp. margarine 1 small orange 1/2 cup nonfat milk Free foods	2 oz. roast beef* 2 slices whole-wheat bread 1 tsp. margarine Mustard to taste 1 medium pickle 1 small apple Free foods	6 oz. orange roughy (baked) 3 oz. tater tots (baked) 7 spears cooked asparagus 1/2 cup nonfat milk Free foods	1 milk exchange 1 fruit exchange Free foods
1,500 calorie menu **ADD to 1,200 menu:**		1 starch/bread exchange 1 vegetable exchange	1 vegetable exchange	1 fruit exchange
1,800 calorie menu **ADD to 1,500 menu:**			1 meat exchange 1 fat exchange	1 fruit exchange 1 fat exchange

*Take roast beef from frozen 1-oz. servings.
Note portion sizes of free foods. Portions beyond these sizes are NOT free!

The Choice Is Yours

DAY 5

Affirmation   The only person who stands in the way of my success is me.

Remember: The benefits of exercise.

Do: DIET: Measure or weigh all food I eat today.
EXERCISE: Do warm-up and cool-down routines.
Practice stretching and flexibility exercises A-1 to A-5.
LIFESTYLE: Spend 15 minutes practicing frustration-control exercises.

Record: Food intake, calories, and fat grams
Calories burned

MENU FOR THE DAY

	Breakfast	Lunch	Dinner	Snack
1,200 calorie menu	1/2 grapefruit 2 slices whole-wheat toast 1 tsp. margarine 2 tsp. sugar-free jelly 1/2 cup egg substitute Free foods	1 cup split pea soup 6 saltines 1 cup nonfat milk 1 cup pears in their own juice 1 cup raw vegetables 2 oz. fat-free cheese Free foods	4 oz. tempeh* stir-fried with 1/2 cup mixed frozen vegetables (nonstarchy) Stir-fry seasoning, as needed 1/3 cup cooked rice Free foods	1 milk exchange 10 peanuts Free foods
1,500 calorie menu **ADD to 1,200 menu:**		1 vegetable exchange	1 vegetable exchange 1 starch/bread exchange	1 fruit exchange
1,800 calorie menu **ADD to 1,500 menu:**			1 meat exchange 1 fat exchange	1 fruit exchange 1 fat exchange

*Tempeh can be purchased in the frozen food section or at a health food store. This soy-based product is an alternative to meat. Excellent taste!
The family will never know what a healthy food you're serving.
Note portion sizes of free foods. Portions beyond these sizes are NOT free!

141

DAY 6

Affirmation: Flexibility is good for my mind as well as my body.

Remember: I must deal with "friendly enemies."

Do: DIET: Follow my menu. Use the "plate method" when choosing my servings.
EXERCISE: Do warm-up and cool-down routines.
Practice stretching and flexibility exercises A-6 to A-10.
LIFESTYLE: Spend 15 minutes practicing motivation exercises.

Record: Food intake, calories, and fat grams
Calories burned

MENU FOR THE DAY

	Breakfast	Lunch	Dinner	Snack
1,200 calorie menu	2/3 cup oatmeal 1 small banana 1/2 cup 4-5% fat cottage cheese 1/2 cup nonfat milk Free foods	2 oz. turkey 2 slices diet bread 1/2 slice (1/2 oz.) fat-free cheese Lettuce leaves 1 Tbsp. reduced-fat mayo Mustard 1 1/4 cups strawberries 1/2 cup nonfat milk Free foods	1 cup spaghetti 1/2 cup meatless nonfat spaghetti sauce Salad greens with fat-free dressing 1 slice Italian bread sprinkled with Italian seasoning "Plate method" requires 1/2 plate of vegetable –green beans it is! Free foods	1 milk exchange 1 fruit exchange Free foods
1,500 calorie menu **ADD to 1,200 menu:**		1 vegetable exchange 1 starch/bread exchange	1 vegetable exchange	1 fruit exchange
1,800 calorie menu **ADD to 1,500 menu:**			1 meat exchange 1 fat exchange	1 fruit exchange 1 fat exchange

Note portion sizes of free foods. Portions beyond these sizes are NOT free!

DAY 7

Affirmation: Giving myself time is not a crime.

Remember: Reward myself for the achievements I have made this week.

Do: DIET: Write my own menu today. Use my favorite foods list.
Replace two high-fat or high-sugar foods with fat-free or sugar-free substitutes.
EXERCISE: Take 20 minutes to relax today.
LIFESTYLE: Share a great joke with someone. Take time for a good hard laugh!

Record: Food intake, calories, and fat grams
Calories burned

MENU FOR THE DAY

	Breakfast	Lunch	Dinner	Snack
1,200 calorie menu	1 milk exchange 1 starch/bread exchange 1 fruit exchange 1 meat exchange 1 fat exchange Free foods	1 starch/bread exchange 1 fruit exchange 2 meat exchanges 1 fat exchange 1 vegetable exchange Free foods	2 starch/bread exchanges 1 fruit exchange 2 meat exchanges 1 fat exchange 1 vegetable exchange Free foods	1 starch/bread exchange 1 milk exchange Free foods
1,500 calorie menu **ADD to 1,200 menu:**		1 starch/bread exchange 1 vegetable exchange	1 vegetable exchange	1 fruit exchange
1,800 calorie menu **ADD to 1,500 menu:**			1 meat exchange 1 fat exchange	1 fruit exchange 1 fat exchange

Note portion sizes of free foods. Portions beyond these sizes are NOT free!

DAY 8

Affirmation: I must not be scared of being prepared.

Remember: Five situations that trigger temptation.

Do: DIET: Plan ahead. Purchase foods I need for this week's menus, including snacks. Allow shopping time to read those labels.

EXERCISE: Do warm-up and cool-down routines.

Do exercises A-1 to A-10. Perform aerobic exercise of my choice for 10 to 20 minutes.

LIFESTYLE: Practice deep-breathing exercise for a minimum of 5 minutes. I need to increase my intensity–push!

Record: Food intake, calories, and fat grams
Calories burned

MENU FOR THE DAY

	Breakfast	Lunch	Dinner	Snack
1,200 calorie menu	1/3 cup Grape-Nuts cereal 1 cup cantaloupe 1/2 cup nonfat milk Free foods	2 oz. chicken 1 small roll 1 (1-oz.) slice fat-free cheese 1 Tbsp. fat-free mayo Pickle slices 1/2 cup nonfat milk Free foods	2 slices meatless pizza Salad greens 1 cup raw vegetables Fat-free dressing 1 cup cantaloupe Free foods	1 fruit exchange 1 vegetable exchange 1 milk exchange Free foods
1,500 calorie menu **ADD to 1,200 menu:**		1 starch/bread exchange 1 vegetable exchange	1 vegetable exchange	1 fruit exchange
1,800 calorie menu **ADD to 1,500 menu:**		1 starch/bread exchange 1 vegetable exchange	1 vegetable exchange 1 meat exchange 1 fat exchange	1 fruit exchange 1 fat exchange

Note portion sizes of free foods. Portions beyond these sizes are NOT free!

DAY 9

Affirmation: I've developed a yearning for calorie burning.

Remember: How aerobic exercise provides more than just calorie consumption.

Do: DIET: Review the favorite foods I have listed. Replace two high-fat or high-sugar foods with fat-free or sugar-free substitutes.

EXERCISE: Do warm-up and cool-down routines. Do exercises A-1 to A-10. Perform aerobic exercise for 10 to 20 minutes.

LIFESTYLE: Spend at least 15 minutes practicing craving-control imagery.

Record: Food intake, calories, and fat grams

Calories burned

MENU FOR THE DAY

	Breakfast	Lunch	Dinner	Snack
1,200 calorie menu	2/3 cup oatmeal 1 small banana 1/4 cup 4-5% fat cottage cheese 1 cup nonfat milk Free foods	1 (1-oz.) slice fat-free lunch meat 2 slices rye bread 1 Tbsp. reduced-fat mayo Lettuce leaves Pickle slices 1 cup cantaloupe Free foods	4 oz. **Poached Fish*** 1 cup steamed carrots 1 medium boiled potato with parsley sprinkles 1 slice angel food cake Free foods	1 milk exchange 1 fruit exchange 15 peanuts Free foods
1,500 calorie menu **ADD to 1,200 menu:**		1 starch/bread exchange 1 vegetable exchange	1 vegetable exchange	1 fruit exchange
1,800 calorie menu **ADD to 1,500 menu:**			1 meat exchange 1 fat exchange	1 fruit exchange 1 fat exchange

* Recipe in Appendix

Note portion sizes of free foods. Portions beyond these sizes are NOT free!

DAY 10

Affirmation: I am managing temptation!

Remember: Three "first responses" that could help me avoid temptation.

Do: DIET: Measure or weigh all food I plan to eat today.
EXERCISE: Do warm-up and cool-down routines. Do exercises A-1 to A-10.
Perform 10 to 20 minutes of aerobic exercise.
LIFESTYLE: Spend at least 15 minutes practicing meditation exercises.

Record: Food intake, calories, and fat grams
Calories burned

MENU FOR THE DAY

	Breakfast	Lunch	Dinner	Snack
1,200 calorie menu	2 slices diet toast 1 tsp. margarine 2 tsp. sugar-free jelly 3/4 cup plain, nonfat yogurt 1/2 cup peaches Free foods	3 oz. water-packed tuna 2 slices diet bread 1 (1-oz.) slice fat-free cheese Lettuce leaves 1 Tbsp. reduced-fat mayo 2 black olives 1/2 grapefruit 1 cup nonfat milk Free foods	**Tofu Chop Suey*** 1 cup white rice Salad greens Fat-free dressing Free foods	1 fruit exchange 1 vegetable exchange Free foods
1,500 calorie menu **ADD to 1,200 menu:**		1 starch/bread exchange 1 vegetable exchange	1 vegetable exchange	1 fruit exchange
1,800 calorie menu **ADD to 1,500 menu:**			1 meat exchange 1 fat exchange	1 fruit exchange 1 fat exchange

* Recipe in Appendix
Note portion sizes of free foods. Portions beyond these sizes are NOT free!

DAY 11

Affirmation: Persistence and resistance will prolong my existence.

Remember: Five ways to continue my diet program when out of town.

Do: DIET: Follow my menu, but use the "plate method" when choosing servings.
EXERCISE: Do warm-up and cool-down routines. Do exercises A-1 to A-10.
Perform 10 to 20 minutes of aerobic exercise.
LIFESTYLE: Spend at least 15 minutes practicing anger-control imagery.

Record: Food intake, calories, and fat grams
Calories burned

MENU FOR THE DAY

	Breakfast	Lunch	Dinner	Snack
1,200 calorie menu	1/4 cup egg substitute 1/2 cup grapefruit sections 1/2 English muffin 1/2 tsp. margarine 2 tsp. sugar-free jelly 1/2 cup nonfat milk Free foods	1 cup vegetable soup 1/4 cup 4-5% fat cottage cheese 1/2 cup peaches (own juice) 14 Wheat Thins 1/2 cup nonfat milk Free foods	4 oz. **No-Fat "Fried" Chicken*** 1 medium baked potato 1 tsp. margarine "Plate Method" requires 1/2 plate of vegetable —broccoli it is! 1/2 cup grapefruit sections Free foods	1 vegetable exchange 1 milk exchange Free foods
1,500 calorie menu **ADD to 1,200 menu:**		1 starch/bread exchange 1 vegetable exchange	1 vegetable exchange	1 fruit exchange
1,800 calorie menu **ADD to 1,500 menu:**			1 meat exchange 1 fat exchange	1 fruit exchange 1 fat exchange

* Recipe in Appendix
Note portion sizes of free foods. Portions beyond these sizes are NOT free!

147

28-Day Guide

DAY 12

Affirmation: Controlling my emotion is a key weight-control notion.

Remember: Three ways to overcome emotional eating.

Do: DIET: Avoid all drinks with calories (sodas, juices, alcoholic beverages), but do not omit my daily 1 cup of nonfat milk.
EXERCISE: Do warm-up and cool-down routines. Do exercises A-1 to A-10. Perform 10 to 20 minutes aerobic exercise.
LIFESTYLE: Spend at least 15 minutes practicing frustration control exercises.

Record: Food intake, calories, and fat grams
Calories burned

MENU FOR THE DAY

	Breakfast	Lunch	Dinner	Snack
1,200 calorie menu	1 slice raisin toast 1 tsp. margarine 1/4 cup egg substitute 1 small orange 1/2 cup nonfat milk Free foods	1/4 cup vegetarian baked beans 1 fat-free hot dog 1 small apple 2 tsp. peanut butter 1 **Oatmeal Raisin Cookie*** 1/2 cup nonfat milk Free foods	4 oz. **Crispy Baked Fish*** 1/2 cup **Oven Broasted Potatoes*** 7 spears steamed asparagus 1 slice angel food cake 1 1/4 cups strawberries Free foods	1 vegetable exchange 1 milk exchange 6 almonds Free foods
1,500 calorie menu **ADD to 1,200 menu:**		1 starch/bread exchange 1 vegetable exchange	1 vegetable exchange	1 fruit exchange
1,800 calorie menu **ADD to 1,500 menu:**			1 meat exchange 1 fat exchange	1 fruit exchange 1 fat exchange

* Recipes in Appendix
Note portion sizes of free foods. Portions beyond these sizes are NOT free!

148

DAY 13

Affirmation: It's not impromptu; I must plan to review.

Remember: Ways to prevent injury when exercising.

Do: DIET: No sweets today. Provide fresh fruit for desserts or snacks.
EXERCISE: Do warm-up and cool-down routines. Do exercises A-1 to A-10.
Perform 10 to 20 minutes of aerobic exercise.
LIFESTYLE: Spend at least 15 minutes practicing motivation exercises.

Record: Food intake, calories, and fat grams
Calories burned

MENU FOR THE DAY

	Breakfast	Lunch	Dinner	Snack
1,200 calorie menu	2 slices **Fat-Free French Toast*** 2 tsp. sugar-free syrup 1 cup cantaloupe Free foods	2 slices diet bread 1 tsp. margarine 1 slice fat-free Swiss cheese 1 cup black bean soup 1 cup cantaloupe ½ cup nonfat milk Free foods	1½ cups **Stovetop Turkey with Noodles*** ½ cup cooked carrots Sugar-free gelatin Free foods	1 fruit exchange 1 milk exchange 9 cashews Free foods
1,500 calorie menu **ADD to 1,200 menu:**		1 starch/bread exchange 1 vegetable exchange	1 vegetable exchange	1 fruit exchange
1,800 calorie menu **ADD to 1,500 menu:**			1 meat exchange 1 fat exchange	1 fruit exchange 1 fat exchange

* Recipe in Appendix
Note portion sizes of free foods. Portions beyond these sizes are NOT free!

DAY 14

Affirmation: Variety makes my exercise sessions more enjoyable.

Remember: Reward myself for my achievements this week.

Do:
DIET: Write my own menu today. Use my favorite foods list.
EXERCISE: Take 20 minutes to relax today.
LIFESTYLE: Share a great joke with someone. Take time for a good hard laugh.

Record: Food intake, calories, and fat grams
Calories burned

MENU FOR THE DAY

	Breakfast	Lunch	Dinner	Snack
1,200 calorie menu	1 milk exchange 1 starch/bread exchange 1 fruit exchange 1 meat exchange 1 fat exchange Free foods	1 starch/bread exchange 1 fruit exchange 2 meat exchanges 1 fat exchange 1 vegetable exchange Free foods	2 starch/bread exchanges 1 fruit exchange 2 meat exchanges 1 fat exchange 1 vegetable exchange Free foods	1 starch/bread exchange 1 milk exchange Free foods
1,500 calorie menu **ADD to 1,200 menu:**		1 starch/bread exchange 1 vegetable exchange	1 vegetable exchange	1 fruit exchange
1,800 calorie menu **ADD to 1,500 menu:**			1 meat exchange 1 fat exchange	1 fruit exchange 1 fat exchange

Note portion sizes of free foods. Portions beyond these sizes are NOT free!

DAY 15

Affirmation: I find strength, not excuses.

Remember: How limiting fat intake can help me achieve my weight goal.

Do: DIET: Purchase foods for this week's menu, including snacks. Take time to read the labels!
EXERCISE: Do warm-up and cool-down routines.
Do exercises B-1 to B-10. Perform 20 to 30 minutes of aerobic exercise.
LIFESTYLE: Practice deep-breathing exercises for at least 7 minutes.

Record: Food intake, calories, and fat grams
Calories burned

MENU FOR THE DAY

	Breakfast	Lunch	Dinner	Snack

1,200 calorie menu	2/3 cup oatmeal
	1 slice **Banana Bread***
	1 small orange
	1/2 cup nonfat milk
	Free foods
		1 fat-free hot dog
		1/4 cup homemade
		   cole slaw
		1 dill pickle
		1 cup raw carrots
		1 frozen fruit bar
		Free foods
			Tempeh Pineapple
			Tomato Pie*
			Salad greens with
			   fat-free dressing
			1 cup mixed raw
			   vegetables
			1/2 cup nonfat milk
			Free foods
				1 milk exchange
				1 fruit exchange
				2 meat exchanges
				Free foods

1,500 calorie menu **ADD to 1,200 menu:**		1 starch/bread exchange 1 vegetable exchange	1 vegetable exchange	1 fruit exchange
1,800 calorie menu **ADD to 1,500 menu:**			1 meat exchange 1 fat exchange	1 fruit exchange 1 fat exchange

* Recipes in Appendix
Note portion sizes of free foods. Portions beyond these sizes are NOT free!

151

DAY 16

Affirmation: My new lifestyle is a matter of perseverance, not persecution.

Remember: All the health benefits of losing weight

Do: DIET: Review the favorite foods I have listed. Replace two high-fat or high-sugar foods with fat-free or sugar-free substitutes.
EXERCISE: Do warm-up and cool-down routines.
Do exercises B-1 to B-10. Perform 20 to 30 minutes of aerobic exercise.
LIFESTYLE: Spend at least 20 minutes practicing meditation exercises.

Record: Food intake, calories, and fat grams
Calories burned

MENU FOR THE DAY

	Breakfast	Lunch	Dinner	Snack
1,200 calorie menu	1 pancake 1 Tbsp. sugar-free syrup 1 cup cantaloupe 1/2 cup 4-5% fat cottage cheese 1/2 cup nonfat milk 1 tsp. margarine Free foods	2 oz. low-fat sandwich meat 2 slices diet bread 1 cup split pea soup 1 cup cantaloupe 1/2 cup nonfat milk Free foods	1 cup **Scalloped Soybeans*** 1/2 cup each of steamed broccoli & cauliflower 1 small dinner roll Free foods	1 fruit exchange 1 milk exchange Free foods
1,500 calorie menu **ADD to 1,200 menu:**		1 starch/bread exchange 1 vegetable exchange	1 vegetable exchange	1 fruit exchange
1,800 calorie menu **ADD to 1,500 menu:**			1 meat exchange 1 fat exchange	1 fruit exchange 1 fat exchange

* Recipe in Appendix
Note portion sizes of free foods. Portions beyond these sizes are NOT free!

The Choice Is Yours

DAY 17

Affirmation: I only get the support I ask for.

Remember: How being an apple or a pear can affect my health.

Do: DIET: Measure or weigh all food I plan to eat today.
EXERCISE: Do warm-up and cool-down routines.
 Do exercises B-1 to B-10. Perform 20 to 30 minutes of aerobic exercise.
 LIFESTYLE: Spend at least 20 minutes practicing meditation exercises.

Record: Food intake, calories, and fat grams
 Calories burned

MENU FOR THE DAY

	Breakfast	Lunch	Dinner	Snack
1,200 calorie menu	1 cup Cheerios cereal 1 cup nonfat milk 1/2 cup fruit cocktail Free foods	1 cup vegetable soup 2 oz. roast beef * 2 slices diet bread 1 cup raw vegetables 1 1/4 cup strawberries 2 Tbsp. whipped topping Free foods	1 3-oz. broiled pork chop 1 medium potato cut in wedges, sprayed with butter flavoring and broiled 1/2 cup cooked broccoli Free foods	1 milk exchange 1 fruit exchange Free foods
1,500 calorie menu **ADD to 1,200 menu:**		1 starch/bread exchange 1 vegetable exchange	1 vegetable exchange	1 fruit exchange
1,800 calorie menu **ADD to 1,500 menu:**			1 meat exchange 1 fat exchange	1 fruit exchange 1 fat exchange

*Take roast beef from frozen 1-oz. servings.
Note portion sizes of free foods. Portions beyond these sizes are NOT free!

DAY 18

Affirmation: I'll take extra precautions in managing my portions.

Remember: Types of fiber that can help improve my health.

Do: DIET: Follow my menu, but use the "plate method" when choosing my servings.
EXERCISE: Do warm-up and cool-down routines.
   Do exercises B-1 to B-10. Perform 20 to 30 minutes of aerobic exercise.
LIFESTYLE: Spend at least 20 minutes practicing anger-control imagery.

Record: Food intake, calories, and fat grams
   Calories burned

MENU FOR THE DAY

	Breakfast	Lunch	Dinner	Snack
1,200 calorie menu	2 frozen low-fat multi-grain waffles 2 Tbsps. sugar-free syrup 1 1/4 cups strawberries 1/2 cup nonfat milk Free foods	1 cup chicken noodle soup 6 saltine crackers 1 cup raw vegetables 1 small pear 1/2 cup nonfat milk 1 frozen fruit bar Free foods	4 oz. roast beef* 1/2 medium boiled potato Salad greens with tomato wedges and fat-free dressing "Plate method" requires 1/2 plate of vegetable —cooked carrots it is! Free foods	1 milk exchange 1 meat exchange Free foods
1,500 calorie menu **ADD to 1,200 menu:**		1 starch/bread exchange 1 vegetable exchange	1 vegetable exchange	1 fruit exchange
1,800 calorie menu **ADD to 1,500 menu:**			1 meat exchange 1 fat exchange	1 fruit exchange 1 fat exchange

*Take roast beef from frozen 1-oz. servings.
Note portion sizes of free foods. Portions beyond these sizes are NOT free!

DAY 19

Affirmation: My genes are not my fault, but my behavior is my responsibility.

Remember: Three ways of overcoming my barriers to weight control.

Do: DIET: Avoid all drinks with calories (soda, juices, alcoholic beverages), but do not omit my daily 1 cup of nonfat milk.
EXERCISE: Do warm-up and cool-down routines. Do exercises B-1 to B-10.
Perform at least 20 minutes of aerobic exercise.
LIFESTYLE: Spend at least 20 minutes practicing frustration-control exercises.

Record: Food intake, calories, and fat grams
Calories burned

MENU FOR THE DAY

	Breakfast	Lunch	Dinner	Snack
1,200 calorie menu	1 **Raisin Bran Muffin*** 1 tsp. margarine 2 tsp. sugar-free jelly 1 small orange 1 cup nonfat milk 1/4 cup 4-5% fat cottage cheese Free foods	1/2 of a 61/2" wheat pita 2-oz. fat-free turkey with Lettuce leaves and Tomato 1 tsp. reduced-fat mayo 1 small banana Free foods	1 serving **Spinach Stuffed Pizza*** Salad greens with 1/2 cup raw vegetables Fat-free dressing 2 small bread sticks Free foods	1 milk exchange 1 fruit exchange 1 vegetable exchange Free foods
1,500 calorie menu ADD to 1,200 menu:		1 starch/bread exchange 1 vegetable exchange	1 vegetable exchange	1 fruit exchange
1,800 calorie menu ADD to 1,500 menu:			1 meat exchange 1 fat exchange	2 fruit exchanges 1 fat exchange

* Recipes in Appendix
Note portion sizes of free foods. Portions beyond these sizes are NOT free!

155

DAY 20

Affirmation: My exercise is motivation in action.

Remember: My reasons for losing weight.

Do: DIET: No sweets today. Provide fresh fruit for desserts or snacks.
EXERCISE: Do warm-up and cool-down routines.
Do exercises B-1 to B-10. Perform 20 to 30 minutes of aerobic exercise.
LIFESTYLE: Spend at least 20 minutes practicing motivation exercises.

Record: Food intake, calories, and fat grams
Calories burned

MENU FOR THE DAY

	Breakfast	Lunch	Dinner	Snack
1,200 calorie menu	1 cup raisin bran cereal 1 cup nonfat milk 1 small orange Free foods	1 cup vegetable soup 2 fat-free hot dogs 1 hot dog bun 1 frozen fruit bar Free foods	3-oz. broiled pork chop 1 cup cooked broccoli 1 tsp. margarine 1 1/4 cups strawberries with 2 Tbsp. whipped topping Free foods	1 milk exchange Free foods
1,500 calorie menu **ADD to 1,200 menu:**		1 starch/bread exchange 1 vegetable exchange	1 vegetable exchange	1 fruit exchange
1,800 calorie menu **ADD to 1,500 menu:**			1 meat exchange 1 fat exchange	1 fruit exchange 1 fat exchange

Note portion sizes of free foods. Portions beyond these sizes are NOT free!

DAY 21

Affirmation: Self-esteem is the barometer of action—the less I do, the more pressure I feel.

Remember: Reward myself for the achievements I have made this week.

Do: DIET: Write my own menu today. Use my favorite foods list.
EXERCISE: Take 20 minutes to relax today.
LIFESTYLE: Share a great joke with someone. Take time for a good hard laugh.

Record: Food intake, calories, and fat grams
Calories burned

MENU FOR THE DAY

	Breakfast	Lunch	Dinner	Snack
1,200 calorie menu	1 milk exchange 1 starch/bread exchange 1 fruit exchange 1 meat exchange 1 fat exchange Free foods	1 starch/bread exchange 1 fruit exchange 2 meat exchanges 1 fat exchange 1 vegetable exchange Free foods	2 starch/bread exchanges 1 fruit exchange 2 meat exchanges 1 fat exchange 1 vegetable exchange Free foods	1 starch/bread exchange 1 milk exchange Free foods
1,500 calorie menu **ADD to 1,200 menu:**		1 vegetable exchange 1 vegetable exchange	1 vegetable exchange	1 fruit exchange
1,800 calorie menu **ADD to 1,500 menu:**			1 meat exchange 1 fat exchange	1 fruit exchange 1 fat exchange

Note portion sizes of free foods. Portions beyond these sizes are NOT free!

DAY 22

Affirmation: Self-control is my antidote to temptation.

Remember: What saturated fat can do to my health.

Do: DIET: Plan and purchase foods for this week's menu, including snacks. Take time to read labels!
EXERCISE: Do warm-up and cool-down routines.
       Do exercises C-1 to C-10. Do aerobic exercise for 30 to 45 minutes.
       LIFESTYLE: Practice deep breathing exercises for 10 minutes.

Record: Food intake, calories, and fat grams
       Calories burned

MENU FOR THE DAY

	Breakfast	Lunch	Dinner	Snack
1,200 calorie menu	3/4 cup Total cereal 1 cup nonfat milk 1/2 cup peach slices Free foods	3 oz. broiled ground round 1 cup cooked broccoli and cauliflower 1/2 cup peach slices Free foods	1 serving (2 pieces) **Cheese Manicotti*** 1/2 cup mixed vegetables 1 slice Italian bread with garlic seasoning 1/2 tsp. margarine Free foods	1 starch/bread exchange 1 milk exchange 1 fruit exchange Free foods
1,500 calorie menu **ADD to 1,200 menu:**		1 starch/bread exchange 1 vegetable exchange	1 vegetable exchange	1 fruit exchange
1,800 calorie menu **ADD to 1,500 menu:**			1 meat exchange 1 fat exchange	1 fruit exchange 1 fat exchange

* Recipe in Appendix
Note portion sizes of free foods. Portions beyond these sizes are NOT free!

DAY 23

Affirmation I enjoy exercising.

Remember: What to look for in a good exercise shoe.

Do: DIET: Review the favorite foods I have listed.
Choose two high-fat or high-sugar foods and replace with fat-free or sugar-free substitutes.
EXERCISE: Do warm-up and cool-down routines. Do exercises C-1 to C-10. Perform aerobic exercise for 30 to 45 minutes.
LIFESTYLE: Spend at least 20 minutes practicing the craving-control imagery.

Record: Food intake, calories, and fat grams
Calories burned

MENU FOR THE DAY

	Breakfast	Lunch	Dinner	Snack
1,200 calorie menu	1 **Raisin Bran Muffin*** 2 tsp. sugar-free jelly 3 prunes 1/4 cup 4-5% fat cottage cheese Free foods	1 oz. sandwich meat 1 slice cheese (1g fat or less) 2 slices rye bread 1/2 cup fruit cocktail 1 cup nonfat milk Free foods	1 3-oz. broiled skinless chicken breast 1/2 cup wild rice 1 cup cooked green beans 1 tsp. margarine Free foods	1 milk exchange 1 fruit exchange Free foods
1,500 calorie menu **ADD to 1,200 menu:**		1 starch/bread exchange 1 vegetable exchange	1 vegetable exchange	1 fruit exchange
1,800 calorie menu **ADD to 1,500 menu:**			1 meat exchange 1 fat exchange	1 fruit exchange 1 fat exchange

Note portion sizes of free foods. Portions beyond these sizes are NOT free!

* Recipe in Appendix

DAY 24

Affirmation: A healthy after-dinner treat is one way of getting my just desserts.

Remember: Four major diseases are caused by obesity.

Do: DIET: Measure or weigh all food I plan to eat today.
EXERCISE: Do warm-up and cool-down routines. Do exercises C-1 to C-10.
Perform 30 to 45 minutes of aerobic exercise.
LIFESTYLE: Spend 30 minutes practicing meditation exercises.

Record: Food intake, calories, and fat grams
Calories burned

MENU FOR THE DAY

	Breakfast	Lunch	Dinner	Snack
1,200 calorie menu	1 pkg. instant plain oatmeal 1 cup plain nonfat, sugar-free yogurt Free foods	1 6½" wheat pita filled with 4 oz. water-packed tuna 1 Tbsp. reduced-fat mayo. ¾ cup mandarin orange slices 1 cup raw vegetables Free foods	4 oz. broiled ham 1 medium baked potato with no-fat butter spray ½ cup cooked carrots 1 cup sugar-free gelatin with ¾ cup mandarin orange slices Free foods	1 milk exchange 1 fruit exchange Free foods
1,500 calorie menu **ADD to 1,200 menu:**		1 starch/bread exchange 1 vegetable exchange	1 vegetable exchange	1 fruit exchange
1,800 calorie menu **ADD to 1,500 menu:**			1 meat exchange 1 fat exchange	1 fruit exchange 1 fat exchange

Note portion sizes of free foods. Portions beyond these sizes are NOT free!

The Choice Is Yours

DAY 25

Affirmation: My belief is more important than my past experiences.

Remember: Three ways to manage stress.

Do: DIET: Follow my menu, but use the "plate method" when choosing my servings.
EXERCISE: Do warm-up and cool-down routines.
Do exercises C-1 to C-10. Perform 30 to 45 minutes of aerobic exercise.
LIFESTYLE: Spend at least 20 minutes practicing anger-control imagery.

Record: Food intake, calories, and fat grams
Calories burned

MENU FOR THE DAY

	Breakfast	Lunch	Dinner	Snack
1,200 calorie menu	2-oz. frozen low-fat multi-grain waffles with ½ tsp. margarine 2 Tbsp. sugar-free syrup ½ cup fruit cocktail 1 cup nonfat milk Free foods	BLT made with 2 slices whole-wheat toast 1 Tbsp. reduced-fat mayo Lettuce leaves, tomato 2 oz. Canadian bacon 1 cup tomato soup made with water Free foods	3-oz. skinless chicken breast, seasoned & baked 1 brown-and-serve roll ½ cup applesauce "Plate method" requires ½ plate of vegetable –frozen broccoli and cauliflower mix it is! Free foods	1 milk exchange 1 fruit exchange Free foods
1,500 calorie menu ADD to 1,200 menu:		1 starch/bread exchange 1 vegetable exchange	1 vegetable exchange	1 fruit exchange
1,800 calorie menu ADD to 1,500 menu:			1 meat exchange 1 fat exchange	1 fruit exchange 1 fat exchange

Note portion sizes of free foods. Portions beyond these sizes are NOT free!

DAY 26

Affirmation: I won't let slip-ups be my downfall.

Remember: How to shake the salt habit.

Do: DIET: Avoid all caloric drinks (soda, juices, alcoholic beverages), but do not omit my daily 1 cup nonfat milk.
EXERCISE: Do warm-up and cool-down routines. Do exercises C-1 to C-10.
Perform aerobic exercise for 30 to 45 minutes.
LIFESTYLE: Spend at least 20 minutes practicing frustration-control exercises.

Record: Food intake, calories, and fat grams
Calories burned

MENU FOR THE DAY

	Breakfast	Lunch	Dinner	Snack
1,200 calorie menu	1 3-oz. whole-grain bagel 1 Tbsp. reduced-fat cream cheese 1 small orange 1/2 cup nonfat milk Free foods	1 fat-free hot dog 1/3 cup vegetarian baked beans 1 small banana 1/2 cup nonfat milk 1 cup raw vegetables Free foods	4 oz. roast pork tenderloin 1/2 cup corn 1/2 cup steamed broccoli 1 small dinner roll 1/2 margarine Sugar-free gelatin Free foods	1 milk exchange 1 fruit exchange Free foods
1,500 calorie menu **ADD to 1,200 menu:**		1 starch/bread exchange 1 vegetable exchange	1 vegetable exchange	1 fruit exchange
1,800 calorie menu **ADD to 1,500 menu:**			1 meat exchange 1 fat exchange	1 fruit exchange 1 fat exchange

Note portion sizes of free foods. Portions beyond these sizes are NOT free!

DAY 27

Affirmation: I will manage fast food by choosing correctly.

Remember: The importance of having someone to support and encourage my efforts.

Do: DIET: No sweets today. Provide fresh fruit for desserts and snacks
        EXERCISE: Do warm-up and cool-down routines.
                 Do exercises C-1 to C-10. Perform 30 to 45 minutes of aerobic exercise.
        LIFESTYLE: Spend 30 minutes practicing motivation exercises.

Record: Food intake, calories, and fat grams
           Calories burned

MENU FOR THE DAY

	Breakfast	Lunch	Dinner	Snack
1,200 calorie menu	3/4 cup Total cereal 1 cup nonfat milk 1/2 cup pineapple chunks Free foods	FAST FOOD! Submarine sandwich from restaurant: 6" roast beef or turkey sandwich without cheese or oil is the wisest choice. Free foods	4 oz. baked cod 1/2 cup noodles 1 tsp. margarine 1/2 cup cooked green beans 1/2 cup homemade cole slaw 1 cup sugar-free gelatin with 1/2 cup pineapple chunks Free foods	1 milk exchange 1 fruit exchange 6 cashews Free foods
1,500 calorie menu **ADD to 1,200 menu:**		1 starch/bread exchange 1 vegetable exchange	1 vegetable exchange	1 fruit exchange
1,800 calorie menu **ADD to 1,500 menu:**			1 meat exchange 1 fat exchange	1 fruit exchange 1 fat exchange

Note portion sizes of free foods. Portions beyond these sizes are NOT free!

DAY 28

Affirmation: I enjoy eating sensibly because I'm improving my health.

Remember: Reward myself for the achievements I have made this week.

Do: DIET: Write my own menu today. Use my favorite foods list.
EXERCISE: Take 20 minutes to relax today.
LIFESTYLE: Share a great joke with someone. Take time for a good hard laugh.

Record: Food intake, calories, and fat grams
Calories burned

MENU FOR THE DAY

	Breakfast	Lunch	Dinner	Snack
1,200 calorie menu	I milk exchange I starch/bread exchange I fruit exchange I meat exchange I fat exchange Free foods	I starch/bread exchange I fruit exchange 2 meat exchanges I fat exchange I vegetable exchange Free foods	2 starch/bread exchanges I fruit exchange 2 meat exchanges I fat exchange I vegetable exchange Free foods	I starch/bread exchange I milk exchange Free foods
1,500 calorie menu **ADD to 1,200 menu:**		I starch/bread exchange I vegetable exchange	I vegetable exchange	I fruit exchange
1,800 calorie menu **ADD to 1,500 menu:**			I meat exchange I fat exchange	I fruit exchange I fat exchange

Note portion sizes of free foods. Portions beyond these sizes are NOT free!

APPENDIX

EXCHANGES FOR COMMON FOODS

Starch/Bread

One starch/bread exchange has:
- 15 grams carbohydrate
- 3 grams protein
- 0 to 1 grams fat
- 80 calories

Breads	Serving size	Exchanges
Bagel	1 (3 oz.)	2 starch/bread
Baking powder biscuit	1	1 starch/bread, 1 fat
Banana bread	1 slice	1 starch/bread, 1 fat
Bread		
Diet (40 cal./slice)	2 slices	1 starch/bread
Italian	1 (3/4" thick) slice	1 starch/bread
Raisin	1 slice	1 starch/bread
White, rye, whole-wheat	1 slice	1 starch/bread
Bread crumbs	3 Tbsp.	1 starch/bread
Breadsticks (8" long, 1/2" wide)	2	1 starch/bread
Brown-and-serve roll	1 (1 oz.)	1 starch/bread
Cereal bars	1	1 1/2 starch/bread, 1 fat
Cinnamon roll with icing	1 medium	1 starch/bread, 1 fat
Cocktail rye bread	3 slices	1 starch/bread
Corn bread	2" square	1 starch/bread, 1 fat
Croissant	1 med.	1 1/2 starch/bread, 2 1/2 fat
Croutons	2/3 cup	1 starch/bread
Dinner roll	1 (1 oz.)	1 starch/bread
English muffin	1	2 starch/bread
French toast	1	1 starch/bread, 1 med-fat meat

Starch/bread: Breads continued...

Hamburger bun . . . . .1 .2 starch/bread
    Diet . . . . .1 . . . . .1 starch/bread

Hard roll .1 . . . . .1 1/2 starch/bread

Hot dog bun . . . . .1 . . . . .2 starch/bread
    Diet . . . . .1 . . . . .1 starch/bread

Melba toast . . . . .5 oblong . . . . .1 starch/bread

Muffin with fruit . . . . .1 small . . . . .1 starch/bread, 1 fat

Pancakes (4" diameter) . . . . .3 . . . . .3 1/2 starch/bread, 1 fat

Pita (6 1/2" diameter) . . . . .1 . . . . .2 starch/bread

Rice cakes . . . . .2 . . . . .1 starch/bread

Shake 'N Bake . . . . .1/4 pouch . . . . .1 starch/bread

Stuffing (prepared) . . . . .1/4 cup . . . . .1 starch/bread, 1 fat

Taco shell . . . . .1 . . . . 1/2 starch/bread, 1/2 fat

Toaster pastry . . . . .1 . . . . .1 starch/bread, 1 1/2 fruit, 1 fat

Tortillas, corn . . . . .1 . . . . .1 starch/bread

Waffle, frozen . . . . .1 (2 oz.) . . . . .1 starch/bread, 1/2 fat

Cereals	Serving size	Exchanges
All-Bran	1/3 cup	1 starch/bread
Apple Raisin Crisp	2/3 cup	1 starch/bread, 1 fruit
Bran Chex	1/2 cup	1 starch/bread
Cheerios	1 cup	1 starch/bread
Cheerios, flavored	1 cup	2 starch/bread
Corn Chex	3/4 cup	1 starch/bread
Corn grits or corn meal	1/2 cup	1 starch/bread
Cream of rice or wheat	1/2 cup	1 starch/bread
Farina	3/4 cup	1 starch/bread
Fruit Muesli	1 cup	2 starch/bread, 2 fruit
Granola	1/4 cup	1 starch/bread
Grape-Nuts	1/3 cup.	2 starch/bread
Oat bran	1/2 cup	1 starch/bread

Starch/bread: Cereals continued…

Oatmeal	2/3 cup	1 starch/bread
Instant, plain	1 packet	1 starch/bread
Instant, flavored	1 packet	2 starch/bread
Puffed wheat	1 1/2 cups	1 starch/bread
Raisin bran	1 cup	2 starch/bread
Shredded wheat	1/2 cup	1 starch/bread
Total	3/4 cup	1 starch/bread
Wheat germ	1/4 cup	1 starch/bread
Wheaties	3/4 cup	1 starch/bread

Crackers	Serving size	Exchanges
Animal crackers	7	1 starch/bread
Cheese-filled	1.5-oz. pkg.	1 1/2 starch/bread, 2 fat
Cheese Nips	20	1 starch/bread, 1 fat
Club	8	1 starch/bread, 1 fat
Goldfish	45	1 starch/bread, 1 fat
Graham crackers (2 1"x1" sq.)	3	1 starch/bread
Harvest Crisps	12	1 starch/bread, 1 fat
Matzo (6" diameter)	1	1 starch/bread
Matzo	3/4 oz.	1 starch/bread
Oyster	27	1 starch/bread
Peanut-butter-filled	6	1 1/2 starch/bread, 1 fat
Ritz	6	1 starch/bread, 1 fat
Rusk	2	1 starch/bread
Ry Krisp	4	1 starch/bread
Saltines	6	1 starch/bread
Sociables	8	1 starch/bread, 1 fat
Teddy Grahams	15	1 starch/bread, 1/2 fat
Town House	8	1 starch/bread, 1 1/2 fat
Triscuits	6	1 starch/bread, 1 fat
Wheat Thins	14	1 starch/bread, 1 fat
Zwieback	2	1 starch/bread

Starch/bread continued...

Pasta/Rice/Potatoes	Serving size	Exchanges
Couscous	1/3 cup	1 starch/bread
Frozen french fries (3 oz.)	small handful	1 1/2 starch/bread, 1 fat
Noodles, cellophane	3/4 cup	1 starch/bread
Noodles, chow mein	1/3 cup	1 starch/bread
Noodles, spaghetti	1/2 cup	1 starch/bread
Potato, baked or boiled	1 med.	2 starch/bread
Potatoes au gratin	1/2 cup	1 1/2 starch/bread, 1/2 fat
Potatoes, mashed	1/2 cup	1 starch/bread
Potato salad	1/2 cup	1 starch/bread, 1 1/2 fat
Rice, fried	1/2 cup	1 starch/bread, 2 fat
Rice, white or brown	1/3 cup	1 starch/bread
Rice, wild	1/2 cup	1 starch/bread
Rice-A-Roni	1/2 cup	2 starch/bread, 1/2 fat
Scalloped potatoes	1/2 cup	1 starch/bread, 1 1/2 fat
Tater Tots	3 oz.	1 starch/bread, 1 fat

Starchy Vegetables	Serving size	Exchanges
Beans (baked, kidney, lima, navy)	1/3 cup	1 starch/bread
Baked, vegetarian	1/2 cup	1 1/2 starch/bread
Black-eyed peas	1/3 cup	1 starch/bread
Corn	1/2 cup	1 starch/bread
Corn, med. ear	1	1 starch/bread
Corn pudding	1/2 cup	1 starch/bread, 1 fat
Eggplant (cooked cubes)	2 cups	1 starch/bread
Miso	3 Tbsp.	1 starch/bread
Mixed vegetables	3/4 cup	1 starch/bread
Onion rings (frozen)	4	1 starch/bread, 2 fat
Peas / lentils	1/3 cup	1 starch/bread
Sweet potato	1/2 med.	1 starch/bread

Starch/bread continued…

Snacks	Serving size	Exchanges
Angel food cake	1/12th cake	1 starch/bread
Bugles	1 oz.	1 starch/bread, 1 fat
Chex Mix	2/3 cup	1 starch/bread, 1 fat
Cookies (in general)	1 (3" diameter)	1 starch/bread, 1 fat
Doritos (15 to 18 chips)	1 oz.	1 starch/bread, 1 fat
Doughnut (no frosting or glaze)	1	1 starch/bread, 1 fat
Fritos (34 chips)	1 oz.	1 starch/bread, 2 fat
Frozen fruit bar	1	1 fruit exchange
Fudgesicle (frozen)	1 bar	1 starch/bread
Gelatin (regular)	1/2 cup	1 starch/bread
Goldfish crackers	45	1 starch/bread, 1 fat
Granola bar (plain)	1	1 starch/bread, 1 fat
Ice cream	1/2 cup	1 starch/bread, 2 fat
Ice milk	1/2 cup	1 starch/bread, 1 fat
Potato chips (15 to 18 chips)	1 oz.	1 starch/bread, 2 fat
Potato chips (lite)	1 oz.	1 starch/bread, 1 fat
Popcorn (made with oil)	3 cups	1 starch/bread, 1 fat
Popcorn (hot-air popped)	5 cups	1 starch/bread
Pretzels	1 oz.	1 1/2 starch/bread
Pudding pop (frozen)	1 bar	1 starch/bread
Sesame sticks	1 oz.	1 starch/bread, 2 fat
Sherbet	1/2 cup	2 starch/bread
Taco / tortilla chips	1 oz.	1 starch/bread, 2 fat
Yogurt (frozen, nonfat)	3/4 cup	2 starch/bread

Meat

In general, one meat exchange is 1 oz. of cooked meat, fish, poultry, or cheese, or 1 egg. Your choices fall into four categories: very lean, lean, medium-fat, and high-fat.

Very Lean Meat

One *very lean* meat exchange has:
- 7 grams protein
- 0 to 1 gram fat
- 35 calories

Very Lean Meat	Serving size	Exchanges
Buffalo	1 oz.	1 meat
Cheese (1 g fat or less)	1 oz.	1 meat
Chicken or turkey, white meat (no skin)	1 oz.	1 meat
Cornish hen (no skin)	1 oz.	1 meat
Egg whites	2	1 meat
Egg substitute	1/4 cup	1 meat
Fish, fresh or frozen	1 oz.	1 meat
Hot dogs (1 g fat or less)	1	1 meat
Sandwich meat (1 g fat or less)	1 oz.	1 meat
Sardines (in spring water)	2	1 meat
Shellfish (lobster, shrimp)	1 oz.	1 meat
Tuna (canned in water)	1 oz.	1 meat

Lean Meat

One *lean* meat exchange has:
- 7 grams protein
- 3 grams fat
- 55 calories

Lean Meat	Serving size	Exchanges
Beef		
Dry, chipped beef	1 oz.	1 meat, 1/2 fat
Flank	1 oz.	1 meat, 1/2 fat

Lean Meat continued...

    Ground round . . . . .1 oz. .1 meat, ^{1}/2 fat

    Roast (rib, chuck, rump) . . . . . . .1 oz. .1 meat, ^{1}/2 fat

    Round .1 oz. .1 meat, ^{1}/2 fat

    Sirloin .1 oz. .1 meat, ^{1}/2 fat

    Steak (T-bone, porterhouse) . . . .1 oz. .1 meat, ^{1}/2 fat

    Stew meat . . . . .1 oz. .1 meat, ^{1}/2 fat

    Sweetbreads . . . . .1 oz. .1 meat, ^{1}/2 fat

    Tenderloin . . . . .1 oz. .1 meat, ^{1}/2 fat

Cheese

    Cheese (3 g fat or less) . . . . . . .1 oz. .1 meat, ^{1}/2 fat

    Cottage cheese (4% to 5% fat) . .^{1}/4 cup . . . . .1 meat, ^{1}/2 fat

    Parmesan (grated) . . . . .2 Tbsp. . . . . .1 meat, ^{1}/2 fat

Fish

    Catfish .1 oz. .1 meat, ^{1}/2 fat

    Herring . . . . .1 oz. .1 meat, ^{1}/2 fat

    Oysters . . . . .6 med. . . . . .1 meat, ^{1}/2 fat

    Salmon (fresh or canned) . . . . . .1 oz. .1 meat, ^{1}/2 fat

    Sardines (in oil) . . . . .2 . . . . .1 meat, ^{1}/2 fat

    Tuna (canned in oil, drained) . . . .1 oz. .1 meat, ^{1}/2 fat

Hot dogs (3 g fat or less) . . . . . . .1 . . . . .1 meat, ^{1}/2 fat

Lamb

    Roast, chop, leg . . . . .1 oz. .1 meat, ^{1}/2 fat

Liver (high in cholesterol) . . . . . . .1 oz. .1 meat, ^{1}/2 fat

Pork

    Canadian bacon . . . . .1 oz. .1 meat, ^{1}/2 fat

    Ham . . . . .1 oz. . . . . .1 meat, ^{1}/2 fat

    Tenderloin, loin chop . . . . .1 oz. .1 meat, ^{1}/2 fat

Lean Meat continued…

Poultry

    Chicken or turkey, dark meat (no skin) . . .1 oz. . . . . .1 meat, ^{1}/$_2$ fat

    Duck or goose (no skin) . . . . .1 oz. . . . . .1 meat, ^{1}/$_2$ fat

Sandwich meat (3 g fat or less) . . . . .1 oz. . . . . .1 meat, ^{1}/$_2$ fat

Veal

    Lean chop, roast . . . . .1 oz. . . . . .1 meat, ^{1}/$_2$ fat

Wild game

    Pheasant . . . . .1 oz. . . . . .1 meat, ^{1}/$_2$ fat

    Rabbit . . . . .1 oz. . . . . .1 meat, ^{1}/$_2$ fat

    Venison . . . . .1 oz. . . . . .1 meat, ^{1}/$_2$ fat

Medium-Fat Meat

One *medium-fat* meat exchange has:
    7 grams protein
    5 grams fat
    75 calories

Medium-Fat Meat	Serving size	Exchanges
Beef		
Corned beef	1 oz.	1 meat, 1 fat
Ground beef	1 oz.	1 meat, 1 fat
Meat loaf	1 oz.	1 meat, 1 fat
"Prime" cuts (such as prime rib)	1 oz.	1 meat, 1 fat
Short ribs	1 oz.	1 meat, 1 fat
Cheese (5 g fat or less)		
Feta	1 oz.	1 meat, 1 fat
Mozzarella	1 oz.	1 meat, 1 fat
Ricotta	^{1}/$_4$ cup	1 meat, 1 fat
String cheese	1 oz.	1 meat, 1 fat

Medium-Fat Meat continued...

Egg (medium) . . . . .1 . . . . .1 meat, 1 fat

Fish

    Any fried fish product . . . . .1 oz. . . . . .1 meat, 2 fat, $^1/2$ starch/bread

    Fish sticks . . . . .4 . . . . .1 meat, 1 starch/bread, 1 fat

Lamb

    Ground lamb patties . . . . .1 oz. . . . . .1 meat, 1 fat

    Rib roast . . . . .1 oz. . . . . .1 meat, 1 fat

Pork

    Boston butt, cutlet . . . . .1 oz. . . . . .1 meat, 1 fat

    Chop . . . . .1 oz. . . . . .1 meat, 1 fat

    Ham salad . . . . .2 Tbsp. .1 meat, 1 fat

    Top loin . . . . .1 oz. . . . . .1 meat, 1 fat

Poultry

    Chicken nuggets . . . . .3 oz. . . . . .2 meat, 1 fat, 1 starch/bread

    Chicken with skin . . . . .1 oz. . . . . .1 meat, 1 fat

    Ground chicken or turkey . . . . .1 oz. . . . . .1 meat, 1 fat

    Turkey bacon . . . . .1 slice . . . . .1 fat

Sausage (5 g fat or less) . . . . .1 oz. . . . . .1 meat, 1 fat

Tempeh (4 oz.) . . . .$^1/4$ cup .1 meat, 1 fat

Tofu (4 oz.) . . . .$^1/2$ cup .1 meat, 1 fat

Veal

    Cutlet .1 oz. . . . . .1 meat, 1 fat

    Ground or cubed . . . . .1 oz. . . . . .1 meat, 1 fat

High-Fat Meat

One *high-fat* meat exchange has:
  7 grams protein
  8 grams fat
  100 calories

High-Fat Meat	Serving size	Exchanges
Bacon	3 slices	1 meat, 1 1/2 fat
Cheese		
American	1 oz.	1 meat, 1 1/2 fat
Cheddar	1 oz.	1 meat, 1 1/2 fat
Monterey Jack, Colby	1 oz.	1 meat, 1 1/2 fat
Gouda, Havarti	1 oz.	1 meat, 1 1/2 fat
Swiss	1 oz.	1 meat, 1 1/2 fat
Falafel	3 patties	1 meat, 1 starch/bread, 2 fat
Peanut butter	2 Tbsp	1 meat, 1 1/2 fat
Pork		
Ground pork	1 oz.	1 meat, 1 1/2 fat
Spare ribs	1 oz.	1 meat, 1 1/2 fat
Sandwich meat (8 g fat or less)		
Bologna	1 oz.	1 meat, 1 1/2 fat
Liver sausage	1 slice	1 meat, 1 1/2 fat
Pimento loaf	1 slice	1 meat, 1 1/2 fat
Salami	1 slice	1 meat, 1 1/2 fat
Sausage		
Brown-and-serve	2 links	1 meat, 3 fat
Brown-and-serve (lite)	2 links	1 meat, 1 1/2 fat
Bratwurst	1	1 meat, 1 1/2 fat
Knockwurst	1	1 meat, 1 1/2 fat
Polish sausage	1	1 meat, 1 1/2 fat
Hot dog (8 g fat or less)	1	1 meat, 1 1/2 fat

Vegetables

One vegetable exchange has:
  5 grams carbohydrate
  2 grams protein
  25 calories

Vegetable	Serving size	Exchanges
Artichoke	$^1/_2$ cup cooked	1 vegetable
Artichoke hearts	$^1/_2$ cup cooked	1 vegetable
Asparagus	7 spears cooked/14 spears raw	1 vegetable
Beans (green, wax, Italian)	$^1/_2$ cup cooked/1 cup raw	1 vegetable
Bean sprouts	$^1/_2$ cup cooked/1 cup raw	1 vegetable
Beets	$^1/_2$ cup cooked/1 cup raw	1 vegetable
Broccoli	$^1/_2$ cup cooked/1 cup raw	1 vegetable
Brussels sprouts	3 sprouts cooked	1 vegetable
Cabbage	$^1/_2$ cup cooked/1 cup raw	1 vegetable
Carrots	$^1/_2$ cup cooked/1 cup raw	1 vegetable
Cauliflower	$^1/_2$ cup cooked/1 cup raw	1 vegetable
Celery	$^1/_2$ cup cooked/1 cup raw	1 vegetable
Cole slaw, homemade	$^1/_2$ cup	1 vegetable
Cucumber	$^1/_2$ cup raw	1 vegetable
Dips		
Jalapeno bean	2 Tbsp.	1 vegetable
Salsa	$^1/_3$ cup	1 vegetable
Taco	$^1/_4$ cup	1 vegetable
Eggplant	$^1/_2$ cup	1 vegetable
Green onions, scallions	$^1/_2$ cup cooked/1 cup raw	1 vegetable
Greens (mustard, kale, collard)	$^1/_2$ cup cooked/1 cup raw	1 vegetable
Kohlrabi	$^1/_2$ cup cooked/1 cup raw	1 vegetable
Leeks	$^1/_2$ cup cooked/1 cup raw	1 vegetable

Vegetables continued...

Lettuce	3 cups	1 vegetable
Mixed vegetables, frozen (no starchy vegetables)	$1/2$ cup	1 vegetable
Mushrooms	$1/2$ cup cooked/1 cup raw	1 vegetable
Okra	$1/2$ cup cooked	1 vegetable
Onions	$1/2$ cup cooked/1 cup raw	1 vegetable
Pea pods	$1/2$ cup cooked/1 cup raw	1 vegetable
Peppers	1 large	1 vegetable
Radishes	$1 1/2$ cups	1 vegetable
Salad greens	3 cups	1 vegetable
Sauerkraut	$1 1/2$ cups	1 vegetable
Spaghetti sauce, meatless, low-fat	$1/2$ cup	2 vegetable
Spinach	$1/2$ cup cooked/1 cup raw	1 vegetable
Summer squash	$1/2$ cup cooked/1 cup raw	1 vegetable
Tomato	$1/2$ cup cooked/1 cup raw	1 vegetable
Tomato juice	$1/2$ cup	1 vegetable
Tomato sauce or paste	2 Tbsp.	1 vegetable
Turnips	$1/2$ cup cooked/1 cup raw	1 vegetable
Water chestnuts	$1/2$ cup cooked	1 vegetable
Zucchini	$1/2$ cup cooked/1 cup raw	1 vegetable

Prepared Vegetable Products	Serving size	Exchanges
Broccoli, cauliflower with cheese sauce	$1/2$ cup	2 vegetable, 1 fat
French-cut green beans with almonds	$1/2$ cup	1 vegetable, $1/2$ fat
Onions in cream sauce	$1/2$ cup	2 vegetable, 1 fat
Vegetables in butter sauce	$1/2$ cup	1 vegetable, $1/2$ fat
V-8 vegetable juice	1 cup	2 vegetable

Fruit

One fruit exchange has:
   15 grams carbohydrate
   60 calories

Fruit	Serving size	Exchanges
Apple	1 small	1 fruit
Apples, dried	4 rings	1 fruit
Applesauce	1/2 cup	1 fruit
Apricot, fresh	4 whole	1 fruit
Apricot, dried	8 halves	1 fruit
Apricot, canned (own juice)	1/2 cup	1 fruit
Banana	5" length	1 fruit
Blackberries, blueberries	3/4 cup	1 fruit
Cantaloupe, small	1/3 melon (1 cup chunks)	1 fruit
Cherries	1/2 cup	1 fruit
Dates	3	1 fruit
Figs	1 1/2	1 fruit
Fruit cocktail (own juice)	1/2 cup	1 fruit
Fruit Roll-Ups (1/2 oz.)	1	1 fruit
Grapefruit	1/2	1 fruit
Grapes	17	1 fruit
Honeydew melon	1 cup cubes	1 fruit
Kiwi	1	1 fruit
Mandarin oranges (own juice)	3/4 cup	1 fruit
Mango, small	1/2	1 fruit
Mixed fruit (own juices)	1/2 cup	1 fruit
Nectarine, small	1	1 fruit
Orange, small	1	1 fruit
Papaya	1/2 fruit	1 fruit
Peach, medium	1	1 fruit

Fruit continued…

Peach, canned (own juice)	$1/2$ cup	1 fruit
Pear, large	$1/2$	1 fruit
Pears, canned (own juice)	$1/2$ cup	1 fruit
Pineapple, fresh	$3/4$ cup	1 fruit
Pineapple, canned (own juice)	$1/2$ cup	1 fruit
Plum, small	1	1 fruit
Prunes	3	1 fruit
Raisins	2 Tbsp.	1 fruit
Strawberries	$1 1/4$ cups	1 fruit
Tangerine	2 small	1 fruit
Watermelon	$1 1/4$ cup cubes	1 fruit

Fruit Juices	Serving size	Exchanges
Apple	$1/2$ cup	1 fruit
Cranberry juice cocktail	$1/3$ cup	1 fruit
Cranberry juice cocktail (lite)	1 cup	1 fruit
Fruit blends	$1/3$ cup	1 fruit
Fruit slush	4 oz.	$1 1/2$ fruit
Fruit tea punch (can)	6 oz.	$1 1/2$ fruit
Grape juice	$1/3$ cup	1 fruit
Grapefruit juice	$1/2$ cup	1 fruit
Lemonade	6 oz.	1 fruit
Orange juice	$1/2$ cup	1 fruit
Pineapple juice	$1/2$ cup	1 fruit
Prune juice	$1/3$ cup	1 fruit
Tang	6 oz.	$1 1/2$ fruit

Milk

Nonfat Milk

One *nonfat* milk exchange has:
- 12 grams carbohydrate
- 8 grams protein
- 0 to 3 grams fat
- 90 calories

Nonfat Milk	Serving size	Exchanges
Nonfat (skim) milk	1 cup	1 milk
Low-fat (1%) milk	1 cup	1 milk
Buttermilk, low-fat	1 cup	1 milk
Chocolate milk, low-fat	1 cup	1 milk, 1 fruit
Evaporated skim milk	1/2 cup	1 milk
Nonfat dry milk	1/3 cup dry	1 milk
Ovaltine with skim milk	1 cup	1 milk, 1 starch/bread
Plain yogurt, nonfat, sugar-free	1 cup	1 milk
Flavored yogurt, nonfat, sugar-free	1 cup	1 milk

Low-Fat Milk

One *low-fat* milk exchange has:
- 12 grams carbohydrate
- 8 grams protein
- 5 grams fat
- 120 calories

Low-Fat Milk	Serving size	Exchanges
Reduced fat (2%) milk	1 cup	1 milk, 1 fat
Plain yogurt, low-fat, sugar-free	3/4 cup	1 milk, 1 fat
Flavored yogurt, low-fat, sugar-free	3/4 cup	1 milk, 1 fat, 1 starch/bread
Soo Moo (soy beverage)	1 cup	1 milk, 1 fat
Sweet acidophilus milk	1 cup	1 milk, 1 fat

Milk continued…

Whole Milk

One *whole* milk exchange has:
- 12 grams carbohydrate
- 8 grams protein
- 8 grams fat
- 150 calories

Whole Milk	Serving size	Exchanges
Whole milk	1 cup	1 milk, 1 1/2 fat
Evaporated whole milk	1/2 cup	1 milk, 1 1/2 fat
Goat's milk	1 cup	1 milk, 1 1/2 fat
Kefir	1 cup	1 milk, 1 1/2 fat
Plain yogurt	1 cup	1 milk, 1 1/2 fat

Fat

One fat exchange (regardless of type) has:
  5 grams fat
  45 calories

Polyunsaturated Fat	Serving size	Exchanges
Margarine (stick, tub, squeeze)	1 tsp.	1 fat
Mayonnaise		
Regular	1 tsp.	1 fat
Reduced fat	1 Tbsp.	1 fat
Nuts, walnuts	4 halves	1 fat
Oil (corn, safflower, soybean)	1 tsp.	1 fat
Salad dressing		
Regular	1 Tbsp.	1 fat
Reduced fat	2 Tbsp.	1 fat
Seeds (pumpkin, sunflower)	1 Tbsp.	1 fat

Monosaturated Fat	Serving size	Exchanges
Avocado	1/8 med.	1 fat
Nuts		
Almonds, cashews	6 nuts	1 fat
Mixed (50% peanuts)	6 nuts	1 fat
Peanuts	10 nuts	1 fat
Pecans	4 halves	1 fat
Oil (canola, olive, peanut)	1 tsp.	1 fat
Olives		
Black	8 large	1 fat
Green, stuffed	10 large	1 fat
Peanut butter	2 tsp.	1 fat
Sesame seeds	1 Tbsp.	1 fat
Tahini paste	2 tsp.	1 fat

Fat continued...

Saturated Fat	Serving size	Exchanges
Bacon	1 slice	1 fat
Bacon grease	1 tsp.	1 fat
Butter		
Stick	1 tsp.	1 fat
Whipped	2 tsp.	1 fat
Reduced fat	1 Tbsp.	1 fat
Chitterlings	2 Tbsp.	1 fat
Coconut	2 Tbsp.	1 fat
Coffee whitener		
Liquid	2 Tbsp.	1 fat
Powder	4 Tbsp.	1 fat
Cream, half-and-half	2 Tbsp.	1 fat
Cream cheese		
Regular	1 Tbsp.	1 fat
Reduced fat (light)	2 Tbsp.	1 fat
Fatback, salt pork, or lard	1 tsp.	1 fat
Gravy		
Canned	1/4 cup	1 fat
From mix	1/2 cup	1 fat
Sour cream		
Regular	2 Tbsp.	1 fat
Reduced fat	3 Tbsp.	1 fat

Combination Foods

Entrees	Serving size	Exchanges
Burrito	1 (6 oz.)	2 starch/bread, 2 meat, 3 fat
Casseroles (tuna noodle, lasagna, spaghetti with meatballs, chili with beans, macaroni and cheese, "Hamburger Helper")	1 cup	2 starch/bread, 2 meat, 2 fat
Chimichangas	1 (6 oz.)	2 starch/bread, 1 meat, 4 fat
Chicken a la King	1 cup	1 starch/bread, 2 meat, 3 fat
Chop suey	1 cup	1 starch/bread, 3 meat, 1 1/2 fat
Chow mein (no noodles or rice)	2 cups	1 starch/bread, 2 meat
French toast	2 slices	2 starch/bread, 2 meat, 3 fat
Pizza, no meat, thin crust	1/4 of 10"	2 starch/bread, 2 meat, 3 fat
Pizza, meat, thin crust	1/4 of 10"	2 starch/bread, 2 meat, 4 fat
Pot pie	1 (7 oz.)	2 starch/bread, 1 meat, 5 fat
Spaghetti sauce, meatless, low-fat	1/2 cup	2 vegetable
Spaghetti sauce with meat	1 cup	4 vegetable, 1/2 meat, 1 fat

Frozen Entrees	Serving size	Exchanges
Chicken Parmigiana	1 (11 oz.)	1 1/2 starch/bread, 1 vegetable, 2 meat, 2 1/2 fat
Macaroni and cheese	1 (8 oz.)	2 1/2 starch/bread, 1 meat, 3 fat
Salisbury steak with gravy and mashed potatoes	1 (11 oz.)	2 starch/bread, 3 meat, 6-7 fat
Turkey with gravy, dressing, and mashed potatoes	1 (11 oz.)	2 starch/bread, 2 meat, 4 fat
Entree with less than 300 calories	1 (8 oz.)	2 starch/bread, 3 meat

Combination Foods continued...

Sandwiches	Serving size	Exchanges
Beef or pork with gravy	1	2 starch/bread, 2 meat, 4 fat
Egg salad	1	2 starch/bread, 1 meat, 3 fat
Grilled cheese	1	2 starch/bread, 2 meat, 4 fat
Ham salad	1	2 starch/bread, 1 meat, 3 fat
Hot dog in bun	1	2 starch/bread, 1 meat, $3^{1}/2$ fat
Peanut butter	1	2 starch/bread, 1 meat, 2 fat
Sub or hoagie	1	4 starch/bread, 4 meat, 5 fat
Tuna salad	1	2 starch/bread, 1 meat, 3 fat

Soups	Serving size	Exchanges
Bean	1 cup	1 starch/bread, 1 meat
Chicken noodle	1 cup	1 starch/bread
Clam chowder (New England style, made with milk)	1 cup	1 starch/bread, 1 fat
Cream of asparagus	1 cup	1 starch/bread, 1 fat
Cup-of-soup		
Broth base	6 oz.	$1/2$ starch/bread
Cream base	6 oz.	$1/2$ starch/bread, 1 fat
Country style	6 oz.	1 starch/bread
Lite	6 oz.	$1/2$ starch/bread
Ramen noodles	1 pkg.	$2^{1}/2$ starch/bread, $1^{1}/2$ fat
Split pea	1 cup	1 starch/bread
Tomato (made with water)	1 cup	1 starch/bread
Vegetable beef	1 cup	1 starch/bread
Vegetarian vegetable	1 cup	1 starch/bread
Won ton (canned)	1 cup	$1/2$ starch/bread

Free Foods

A free food is any food or drink with less than 20 calories per serving.

Food

Candy, hard, sugar-free (1 piece)

Chewing gum (2 pieces)

Cream cheese, fat-free (1 Tbsp.)

Creamers, nondairy, liquid (1 Tbsp.)

Creamers, nondairy, powder (2 tsp.)

Dips

    Lean cream dip (1 Tbsp.)

    Picante sauce (2 Tbsp.)

Frozen desserts

    Sugar-free Popsicle (1)

    Crystal Lite bar (1)

Gelatin, sugar-free

Gravies

    Au jus (1/4 cup)

    All others (2 Tbsp.)

Jam or jelly, low-sugar or lite (2 tsp.)

Margarine, fat-free (4 Tbsp.)

Margarine, reduced fat (1 tsp.)

Mayonnaise, fat-free (1 Tbsp.)

Mayonnaise, reduced fat (1 tsp.)

Miracle Whip, fat-free (1 Tbsp.)

Miracle Whip, reduced fat (1 tsp.)

Nonstick cooking spray

Salad dressing, fat-free (1 Tbsp.)

Salsa (1/4 cup)

Sour cream, fat-free (1 Tbsp.)

Syrup, sugar-free (2 Tbsp.)

Whipped topping, regular or lite (2 Tbsp.)

Drinks

Bouillon broth

Carbonated water or mineral water

Cocoa powder, sugar-free

Coffee

Club soda

Diet soda

Drink mixes, sugar-free

Tea

Tonic water

Free Foods continued on next page...

Free Foods continued...

Condiments

Bac-Os (1 tsp.)	Mustard
Barbecue sauce (1 Tbsp.)	Pickles, dill (1 1/2 large)
Catsup (1 Tbsp.)	Soy sauce
Horseradish	Taco sauce
Lemon juice	Vinegar
Lime juice	

Seasonings

Flavoring extracts	Spices
Garlic	Stir-fry seasonings
Herbs	Tabasco
Italian seasoning mix	Wine, used in cooking
Pimento	Worcestershire sauce

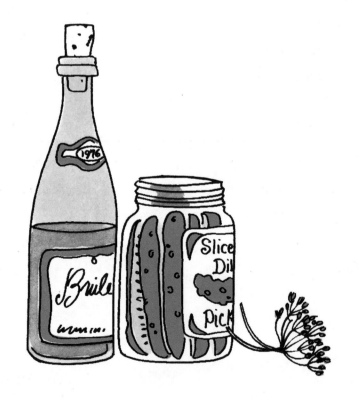

RECIPES

The following recipes are included in the menu plans of the 28-day guide.

Poached Fish

4 servings

1$\frac{1}{2}$ cups chicken broth

1 medium onion, chopped

1 tsp. lemon juice

1 Tbsp. dried parsley

1 bay leaf

1 lb. cod filets

Combine broth, onion, lemon juice, parsley, and bay leaf. Bring to a boil. Place fish in boiling liquid. Reduce heat to low. Cover pan. Simmer until fish flakes easily when slightly lifted with fork (about 8 to 10 minutes). Using slotted spoon, carefully lift fish to serving plate.

Per serving (3$\frac{1}{2}$ oz.): 115 calories, 25 g protein, 1 g carbohydrate, 1 g total fat, trace saturated fat, 55 mg cholesterol, 0.2 g dietary fiber, 188 mg sodium
EXCHANGES: 3 lean meat

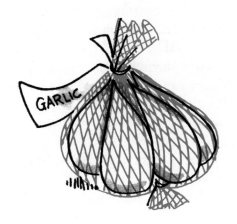

Tofu Chop Suey

4 servings

Tofu tastes like chicken in this recipe!

8 oz. tofu (low-fat)

2 tsp. olive oil

1 Tbsp. minced fresh ginger (available in produce dept.)

1 Tbsp. minced fresh garlic

1 medium onion, chopped

1 cup chopped celery

$\frac{1}{4}$ red bell pepper, seeded and chopped

$\frac{1}{4}$ green bell pepper, seeded and chopped

1$\frac{1}{2}$ cups bean sprouts

$\frac{1}{2}$ cup chicken broth or bouillon

1 Tbsp. soy sauce

Salt (optional) and pepper to taste

1 cup cooked white rice

Drain tofu. Dice into $\frac{3}{4}$-inch cubes. Place cubes between layers of paper toweling; place dinner plate atop pile to weigh it down. Let stand 10 minutes to compress cubes and remove excess water. Heat olive oil in wok or frying pan. Add ginger, garlic, onion, celery, and red and green pepper. Stir-fry over medium-high heat for 1 to 2 minutes. Add bean sprouts, broth, soy sauce, and diced tofu. Stir-fry until vegetables are crisp-tender and liquid has cooked away. Season to taste with salt (optional) and pepper. Serve over cooked white rice.

Per serving (1 cup): 135 calories, 10 g protein, 7 g carbohydrate, 7 g total fat, trace cholesterol, 2.4 g dietary fiber, 45 mg sodium
EXCHANGES: 1 meat, 1 vegetable, $\frac{1}{2}$ fat, 3 starch/bread

No-Fat "Fried" Chicken
4 servings

3 Tbsp. grated Parmesan cheese
1/2 cup bread crumbs
1/2 tsp. rosemary
1/2 tsp. thyme
1 clove garlic, minced
1/4 tsp. onion powder
2 egg whites
4 small skinless chicken breasts

Preheat oven to 400°F. Spray pan with nonstick cooking spray. Combine all ingredients except egg whites and chicken. Beat egg whites; dip chicken breasts into beaten egg whites, then roll them in mixture of dry ingredients. Bake 30 to 40 minutes until done.

Per serving (1 small breast): 183 calories, 32 g protein, 5 g carbohydrate, 3 g total fat, 45 g cholesterol, 313 mg sodium
EXCHANGES: 3 meat, trace fat

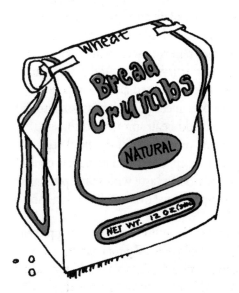

Crispy Baked Fish
4 servings

1 lb. fresh fish (Note: tail portions have fewer bones)
2 Tbsp. fat-free "creamy" salad dressing
1/2 cup bread crumbs

Coat fish with salad dressing. Roll in bread crumbs. Place fish on baking sheet coated with cooking spray.
Bake at 425°F for 10 to 12 minutes.

Per serving (3 1/2 oz.): 125 calories, 25 g protein, 4 g carbohydrate, 1 g total fat, trace saturated fat, 55 mg cholesterol, 0.1 g dietary fiber, 175 mg sodium
EXCHANGES: 3 lean meat

Oven Broasted Potatoes
4 servings

4 medium potatoes
Cooking spray (any brand)

Wash potatoes and cut into wedges. Spray on all sides with cooking spray. Place in single layer on cookie sheet. Bake at 475°F for 35 minutes.

In a hurry? Microwave whole potatoes for approximately 4 minutes. Cut into wedges and spray with cooking spray. Place on cookie sheet and broil until brown.

Per serving (1 potato): 80 calories, 15 g carbohydrate, 3 g protein, trace fat
EXCHANGES: 1 starch/bread

Oatmeal Raisin Cookies
36 cookies

1/3 cup brown sugar or Sugar Twin brown
    sugar substitute
1/4 cup apple juice concentrate
2/3 cup soft margarine
2 eggs or 1/2 cup liquid egg substitute
1 tsp. baking soda
1/2 tsp. salt
1/2 tsp. cinnamon
1 tsp. vanilla
1/2 tsp. nutmeg
1 1/2 cups flour
1 1/2 cups quick oats
2/3 cup raisins

Preheat oven to 350°F. In large mixing
bowl, beat brown sugar, apple juice
concentrate, and margarine until creamy.
Add eggs and mix well. In separate bowl,
mix baking soda, salt, cinnamon, vanilla,
and nutmeg. Add to creamed mixture and
blend. Fold in flour, oats, and raisins.
Drop spoonfuls onto nonstick baking
sheet and bake for about 12 minutes.

Per serving (1 cookie): 60 calories (53 calories
    with sugar substitute), 1 g protein,
    10 g carbohydrate (8 g with sugar
    substitute), 2 g total fat, 12 mg cholesterol
    (0 cholesterol with egg substitute),
    94 mg sodium
EXCHANGES: 1 starch/bread

Stovetop Turkey with Noodles
4 servings

1 cup white sauce (recipe below)
4 oz. (dry) bow-tie noodles, cooked
    according to package directions
2 cups turkey, cooked and cubed
2 cups frozen sugar snap peas, thawed

Prepare white sauce. Add noodles, turkey,
and snap peas. Heat through.

Per serving (1 1/2 cups): 155 calories,
    16 g protein, 16 g carbohydrate,
    2.5 g total fat, <50 mg cholesterol
EXCHANGES: 1 starch/bread, 2 meat,
    1 vegetable, 1/2 fat

White Sauce

2 Tbsp. margarine
2 Tbsp. flour
1 tsp. chicken soup base (or one bouillon
    cube dissolved in water)
1 cup nonfat milk

In saucepan, melt margarine. Remove
from heat and add other ingredients.
Return to medium heat and stir constantly
until mixture thickens.

Fat-Free French Toast
4 servings

1 whole medium egg
2 egg whites
1/2 tsp. vanilla
1/2 cup nonfat milk
8 slices bread

With fork or wire whip, whip together whole egg, egg whites, vanilla, and milk until well blended. Coat frying pan with cooking spray; heat to medium high. Dip bread slices into egg mixture and place in pan. Brown both sides of bread. Top with low-calorie syrup or fruit (calories/exchanges not included).

Per serving (2 slices): 193 calories,
    4 g protein, 30 g carbohydrate,
    5 g total fat, 137 mg cholesterol
    when made with eggs (0 g with egg
    substitute), 358 mg sodium
EXCHANGES: 2 starch/bread, 1/2 meat,
    1/2 milk, trace of fat

Tempeh Pineapple Tomato Pie
4 servings

1 Tbsp. oil
1 small onion, coarsely chopped
8 oz. tempeh, crumbled
1 cup pineapple chunks
1 1/2 cups pizza sauce
12-inch pizza crust

Preheat oven to 400°F. In large skillet, heat oil over low heat. Add onion; saute for 2 minutes. Add tempeh; cook for about 15 minutes. Add pineapple chunks. Mix thoroughly. Spread pizza sauce over pizza crust. Top with tempeh mixture. Bake for about 15 minutes or until crust is browned and sauce is bubbly.

Per serving (1/4 pie): 310 calories,
    15 g protein, 43 g carbohydrate,
    9 g total fat, trace cholesterol
EXCHANGES: 2 meat, 2 fat,
    3 starch/bread

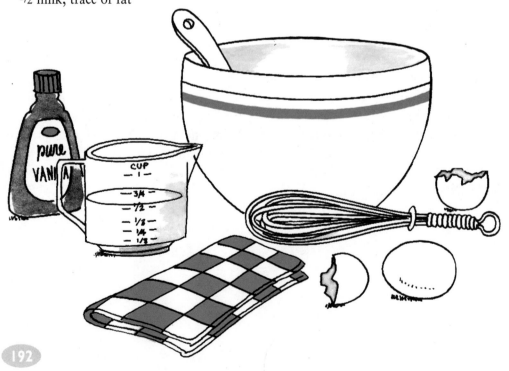

Banana Bread
14 servings

$1^1/2$ cups whole-wheat flour
$1/2$ cup unsweetened shredded coconut
2 tsp. baking powder
$1/2$ tsp. baking soda
$1/2$ tsp. salt (optional)
1 cup mashed ripe (or overripe) banana
3 Tbsp. vegetable oil
2 Tbsp. honey

Preheat oven to 350°F. Lightly grease an 8″ x 4″ loaf pan, or coat pan with vegetable spray. In mixing bowl, combine flour, coconut, baking powder, baking soda, and salt (optional). In another mixing bowl, combine banana, oil, and honey. Stir banana mixture into dry ingredients until just combined; do not overmix. Batter should be lumpy and stiff. Spread batter evenly into prepared loaf pan. Bake until toothpick inserted into the center comes out clean (about 45 to 50 minutes). Allow banana bread to cool in the pan about 10 minutes, then turn bread out of pan and cool completely on rack.

Per serving ($1^1/2$″-thick slice): 112 calories, 2 g protein, 13 g carbohydrate, 5 g total fat, trace cholesterol, 2.1 g dietary fiber, 168 mg sodium (or 92 mg if salt is omitted)
EXCHANGES: 1 starch/bread, 1 fat

Scalloped Soybeans
4 servings

1 cup soybeans, soaked overnight and drained
3 cups water
$1/2$ cup chopped onions
1 cup chopped celery
$1/2$ red bell pepper, seeded and sliced
$1/2$ green bell pepper, seeded and sliced
$1/2$ cup tomato sauce
$1/2$ cup chopped fresh Italian tomato
$1/2$ tsp. salt
$1/4$ cup boiling water
$1/4$ cup bread crumbs
$1^1/2$ tsp. margarine

Place soybeans in saucepan with 3 cups of water. Bring to boil; boil 10 minutes. Lower heat, cover, and simmer $1^1/2$ to 2 hours or until soybeans are softened. Drain. Preheat oven to 350°F. In 6-cup casserole, combine cooked soybeans, onion, celery, red and green peppers, tomato sauce, chopped tomatoes, salt (optional), and $1/4$ cup boiling water. Blend bread crumbs and margarine; sprinkle over soybean mixture. Bake $1^1/2$ to 2 hours.

Per serving (1 cup): 198 calories, 12 g protein, 16 g carbohydrates, 9 g total fat, 1 g saturated fat, trace cholesterol, 5.2 g dietary fiber, 513 mg sodium (or 246 mg if salt is omitted)
EXCHANGES: 1 starch/bread, 1 lean meat, 1 fat

Raisin Bran Muffin
12 muffins

1 1/4 cups all-purpose flour
1/2 cup sugar
1 Tbsp. baking powder
1/4 tsp. salt
2 cups bran cereal
1 cup nonfat milk
1/4 cup nonfat vanilla creamer
1/4 cup unsweetened applesauce
1/2 cup raisins
Vegetable cooking spray

Stir together flour, sugar, baking powder, and salt. Set aside. In large mixing bowl, combine cereal, milk, and creamer. Let stand about 5 minutes or until cereal softens. Add applesauce. Beat well. Add flour mixture and raisins, stirring only until combined. Spray twelve 2 1/2″ muffin cups with cooking spray. Pour batter into muffin cups. Bake at 400°F for approximately 20 minutes or until lightly browned.

Per serving (1 muffin): 130 calories,
    3 g protein, 32 g carbohydrates,
    trace total fat, 5 g dietary fiber
EXCHANGES: 1/3 meat, 2 starch/bread,
    trace fat

Cheese Manicotti
4 servings

8 pieces manicotti
1 cup low-fat (1%) cottage cheese
1/2 cup Parmesan cheese
1 cup prepared spaghetti sauce
    (original flavor)

Cook manicotti according to package directions. Cool. Mix cheeses.
Divide evenly and stuff into each manicotti. Place in microwave-safe baking dish. Pour spaghetti sauce over manicotti. Cover. Microwave on high for 5 minutes or until heated through.

Per serving (2 pieces): 266 calories,
    16 g protein, 35 g carbohydrates,
    5 g total fat, <50 mg cholesterol,
    1 g dietary fiber
EXCHANGES: 2 meat, 2 starch/bread,
    1 fat

Spinach Stuffed Pizza
4 servings

1 package boxed pizza crust mix
1 cup low-fat (1%) cottage cheese
1/2 cup Parmesan cheese
1 10-oz. package frozen spinach, thawed, with excess liquid pressed out
1/2 cup canned pizza sauce

Mix pizza crust according to package directions. Roll out two-thirds of pizza dough and place in deep 9" pie plate. Bake according to package instructions until lightly browned. Mix cottage cheese, Parmesan cheese, and spinach. Spread over crust. Roll out remaining pizza crust and place on top of spinach mixture. Top with pizza sauce. If desired, add mushrooms or onions on top of sauce. (To enhance appearance, sprinkle with 1 Tbsp. Parmesan cheese.) Bake according to crust package instructions until pizza is heated through and crust is browned.

Per serving (1/4 pizza): 300 calories, 13 g protein, 10 g carbohydrate, 6 g total fat, <50 mg cholesterol, 3 g dietary fiber
EXCHANGES: 1 1/2 meat, 3/4 starch/bread, 1 fat

Lifestyle, not "diet"–that's our goal! A healthy lifestyle requires some diversity. Although the following recipes are not referred to in the 28-day guide, you might like to try them to give ethnic variety to your menus.

No-Fry Tortilla Chips
Corn Tortilla Chips
12 servings
Flour Tortilla Chips
24 servings

12 6" corn tortillas, OR 12 10" flour tortillas
warm water
salt (optional)

Immerse tortillas one at a time in warm water. Let drain briefly, then lay flat. If desired, sprinkle lightly with salt. Cut each flour tortilla into eight wedges, or each corn tortilla into six wedges. Place single layer of wedges, salt side up, on nonstick baking sheet or pan. Place wedges close together but do not overlap. Bake at 500°F for 4 minutes. Turn with spatula, then continue to bake until golden brown and crisp–another 3 minutes for corn tortillas and 1 minute for flour tortillas. Cool. Store in airtight bag.

Corn Tortilla Chips
Per serving (1/2 cup or 1 tortilla): 49 calories, 2 g protein, 9 g carbohydrate, 0.8 g total fat, 0.7 g fiber, 39 mg sodium
EXCHANGES: 1/2 starch/bread

Flour Tortilla Chips
Per serving (1/2 cup or 1/2 tortilla): 87 calories, 2 g protein, 16 g carbohydrate, 1.6 g total fat, 0.7 g fiber
EXCHANGES: 1 starch/bread

Frijoles De La Olla
(Boiled Mexican Beans)
10 servings

1 lb. dried pinto beans*
1 medium onion, peeled, diced
5 cups water
1 tsp. salt

Rinse beans and clean of debris.
Place beans and onion in large pot with
water. Cover and simmer over low heat
for at least 2½ hours, or cook overnight
in a slow-cooker such as a crock pot.
Add salt after beans are cooked.

*Beans do not need to be soaked
  before cooking.

Per serving (²/₃ cup): 161 calories,
  10 g protein, 30 g carbohydrate,
  0.6 g total fat, 9.1 g fiber, 219 mg
  sodium
EXCHANGES: 2 starch/bread

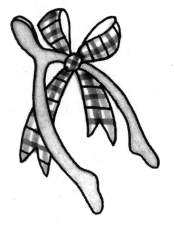

Chicken Caldo
14 servings

1 whole 3-lb. chicken, skinned
1 large onion, chopped
2 to 3 cloves garlic, minced
2 quarts water
1 stalk celery, sliced
1 medium turnip, peeled and cut
  into ½" cubes
2 medium carrots, sliced
2 medium zucchini, sliced
1 15-oz. can kidney beans or hominy,
  drained
1 small head cabbage, chopped
2 tsp. salt
¼ tsp. black pepper

Place chicken, onion, and garlic in large
saucepan or Dutch oven. Cover with
water. Bring to boil. Reduce heat; simmer
for 50 to 60 minutes or until chicken is
tender. Remove chicken from broth and
cool. Take meat from bones. Skim fat
from broth, then return meat to pan.
Add remaining ingredients. Simmer for 20
to 30 minutes or until vegetables are tender.

Per serving (1 cup): 108 calories,
  12 g protein, 10 g carbohydrate, 3 g total
  fat, 27 mg cholesterol, 4 g fiber, 353 mg
  sodium
EXCHANGES: 1 meat, 2 vegetable

CHEF'S TIPS AND RECIPES

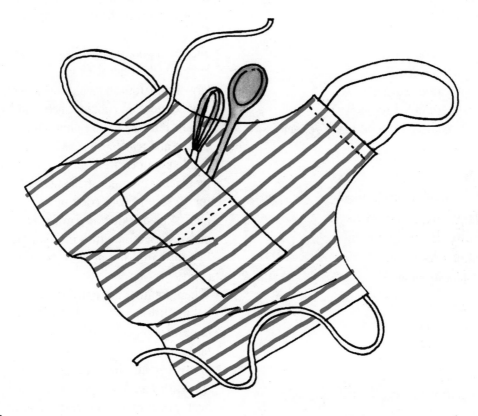

Something special

Beginning a new lifestyle also involves being prepared for special occasions. To assist your efforts, we consulted chef Karla Fischer.

Chef Karla has created some innovative recipes and included cooking tips especially for TOPS members. Enjoy!

Chef's special recipes

This is a new lifestyle for you—not a diet! Therefore, you will certainly have special occasions when you will want to share this healthy lifestyle with others. We hope these healthy and exciting new recipes will soon become some of your favorites.

Herb and Lemon Baked Rainbow Trout with Rosemary Potatoes, Cucumbers, Onion, and Tomatoes

4 servings

Ingredients

Potatoes

3 cups new potatoes, skins on
2 Tbsp. butter
1/2 tsp. paprika
1/2 tsp. onion powder
1/2 tsp. dill weed
1/2 tsp. garlic powder
1/2 tsp. crumbled rosemary
1/8 tsp. coarsely ground black pepper
Pinch of salt

Fish

4 6-oz. rainbow trout filets
2 Tbsp. chopped fresh chives
2 Tbsp. chopped fresh dill
Zest of 1 lemon
1/2 tsp. seasoning salt

Cucumber

1 cup sliced onion
1/2 tsp. white vinegar
1 large cucumber, peeled, seeded, and diced
1 large ripe tomato, seeded, skinned, and diced
2 Tbsp. fresh dill

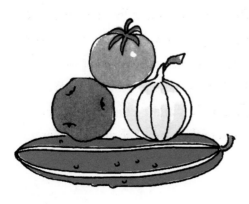

Assembly

- Start potatoes first.
- Boil potatoes about 10 minutes until cooked halfway through but still firm. Drain and cool.
- Slice each potato in half (or in fourths if large). Melt butter with seasonings in large bowl. Toss all ingredients together. Lay potatoes on cooking sheet and bake at 450°F for 25 to 30 minutes until brown and tender.
- While potatoes are boiling, prepare fish by placing on a nonstick sheet sprayed for 1/2 second with cooking spray. Lay filets skin-side-down. Top with herbs and zest. Season with salt. Spray tops of fish for half a second with cooking spray.
- When potatoes are halfway done, begin baking fish in oven at 450°F for 8 to 10 minutes and begin cooking cucumber mixture.
- Spray a small saucepan with cooking spray for half a second. Over very low heat, sweat onions in white vinegar until translucent. Add cucumbers. Continue cooking until soft. Add tomato and dill.

Presentation

- Place fish filet on plate and top with cucumber mixture.
- Serve with rosemary potatoes.

Per serving: 464 calories, 40 g protein, 49 g carbohydrate, 12 g total fat, 5 g fiber, 387 mg sodium
EXCHANGES: 1 vegetable, 3 starch/bread, 5 meat, 1 fat

Broiled Chicken Breast with
Red-Wine-Poached Mushrooms and Leeks
Roasted Garlic Mashed Potatoes
Honey-Glazed Carrots

4 servings

Ingredients
Chicken

4 4-oz. skinless, boneless chicken breasts
1/2 tsp. seasoned salt

Sauce

1 cup chopped leeks
1 clove garlic
1/4 cup cabernet sauvignon
2 1/2 cups sliced mushrooms

Potatoes

3 large Idaho potatoes
2 bulbs garlic wrapped in foil and
   roasted 1 hour at 400°F
1/4 cup skim milk
1/4 tsp. ground rosemary
Dash of nutmeg
1 Tbsp. butter

Carrots

1 Tbsp. honey
2 Tbsp. butter
Pinch of salt
Pinch of white pepper
2 cups sliced carrots, steamed or boiled until
   tender-crisp

Assembly

- Chicken: Preheat broiler. Season
  chicken breasts with seasoned salt. Broil
  3 to 4 minutes per side.
- Sauce: Cover leeks and garlic with

wine. Simmer 5 minutes. Add mushrooms and continue to simmer until
soft (5 more minutes). Keep warm.

- Potatoes: Peel and chop potatoes. Cover
  in water and simmer about 20 minutes,
  or until soft. Meanwhile, place rest of
  potato ingredients in mixer bowl. Drain
  potatoes and mash or mix with rest of
  ingredients. Cover to keep warm.
- Carrots: Combine honey, butter, salt,
  and pepper. Mix together and heat until
  the mixture forms into a glaze. Add
  carrots and lightly toss until coated.

Presentation

- Place one chicken breast on each plate.
- Divide sauce over each plate.
- Serve with scoop of garlic-mashed pota-
  toes and honey-glazed carrots.

Per serving: 535 calories, 45 g protein,
   55 g carbohydrate, 15 g total fat, 5 g
   fiber, 248 mg sodium
EXCHANGES: 4 vegetable, 2 starch/bread,
   5 meat, 2 fat

Spicy Chicken Breast with
Orange Red Onion and Roasted Pepper Relish
Parmesan Green Beans
Orange/Cilantro Rice

4 servings

Ingredients
Dry Seasoning Mix

1 tsp. each of the following:
  Salt
  Onion powder
  Cayenne pepper
  Thyme leaves
  Garlic powder
  Paprika

Relish

2 large oranges, peeled and sectioned, pith and seeds removed, chopped (zest oranges before peeling and reserve for the rice)

2 large red bell peppers, roasted, peeled, seeded, and chopped

1 large red onion, diced

4 Tbsp. chopped fresh cilantro

1 Tbsp. balsamic vinegar

4 basil leaves, chopped

1/4 tsp. ground cumin

1/8 tsp. crushed red pepper flakes

Rice

1 cup dry parboiled rice

2 cups water

1 clove garlic, minced

Zest of two oranges, chopped

1/2 cup chopped cilantro

Other

1 Tbsp. olive oil

4 4-oz. skinless, boneless chicken breasts

4 cups fresh green beans

4 Tbsp. Parmesan cheese

Assembly

- Prepare dry seasoning mix. Set aside.
- Prepare relish. Set aside and leave at room temperature.
- Prepare rice by placing it in water with garlic and orange zest. Cook according to rice package directions.
- Sprinkle dry seasoning over the four chicken breasts.
- Heat olive oil in nonstick saute pan.
- Saute chicken on both sides, lowering heat after turning, about 4 minutes per side, until done but still juicy.
- Steam green beans.
- Add cilantro to rice just before serving.

Presentation

- Divide rice among 4 plates.
- Place 1 chicken breast atop rice and cover with relish.
- Serve with green beans sprinkled with Parmesan cheese.

Per serving: 425 calories, 45 g protein, 37 g carbohydrate, 11 g total fat, 5 g fiber, 214 mg sodium
EXCHANGES: 3 vegetable, 1 fruit, 1 starch/bread, 2 meat, 1 fat

Cod en Papilotte
Gingered Vegetables and Lime
Jasmine Rice

4 servings

Ingredients
Fish
4 6-oz. cod filets
1/4 cup chopped cilantro
Salt and pepper to taste

Vegetables
1 clove garlic, chopped
1/8 cup grated ginger root
1 Tbsp. sesame oil
1 Tbsp. butter
1 small carrot, julienned
1 onion, sliced
3 stalks celery, julienned
4 mushrooms, sliced
1/2 cup roughly chopped pea pods
1/2 cucumber, peeled and sliced

Rice
1 cup cooked jasmine rice

Other
4 large pieces (12″ x 16″) parchment paper (Available at cooking supply stores. You can substitute aluminum foil if paper is not available.)
1 lime, cut in wedges

Assembly
- Saute garlic and ginger in sesame oil and butter for 2 minutes.
- In large bowl, toss vegetables with garlic/butter/ginger mixture. Coat well.
- Fold each piece of parchment in half, folding across the middle of the long side.
- Cut a half-circle with the fold being the straight side.
- Open each circle of paper and place one piece of cod on the bottom half. Sprinkle each with salt and pepper and 1 Tbsp. chopped cilantro.
- Divide the vegetables equally among the four packages.
- Fold top of paper back over cod.
- Make 2″ folds, beginning at the ends, starting each new fold halfway through the last fold.
- After you reach the top, place the package on a sheet pan and bake at 450°F for 15 minutes.

Presentation
Serve each package with lime wedges and 1/4 cup cooked jasmine rice per serving.

Per serving: 228 calories, 33 g protein, 20 g carbohydrate, 8 g total fat, 2 g fiber, 184 mg sodium
EXCHANGES: 1 vegetable, 1 starch/bread, 4 meat, 1 fat

Grilled Chicken Breast with Roasted Red Pepper Coulis
Gremolata
Basmati Rice
Asparagus

4 servings

Ingredients
Chicken
4 4-oz. skinless, boneless chicken breasts
$1/2$ tsp seasoned salt

Coulis
2 medium red bell peppers

Gremolata
$1/2$ cup chopped fresh parsley
2 cloves fresh garlic, finely chopped
Zest of 2 lemons, finely chopped

Other
$2/3$ cup dry basmati rice
1 lb. fresh asparagus
Cooking spray

Assembly
- Trim any fat off chicken breasts. Pound lightly with meat mallet. Season breasts in seasoning salt. Refrigerate.
- To prepare coulis: Over a gas flame or under a broiler, char the red peppers on all sides until blackened. Place in a paper bag, seal, and let steam 10 minutes. Rinse off blackened skin. Remove seeds and stem. Place in food processor or blender and puree until smooth. Set aside.
- To prepare gremolata: Combine parsley, garlic, and lemon zest. Cover and set aside.
- Cook rice in $1/3$ cup water until fluffy. Keep warm.
- Steam asparagus.
- On preheated grill that has been covered with aluminum foil and sprayed with cooking spray for $1/2$ second, cook chicken breasts about 3 minutes per side or until done but still juicy.
Note: The chicken is much more flavorful when cooked on a grill, but you may broil or poach it instead.

Presentation
- Divide rice on four plates.
- Place one chicken breast atop rice and drizzle with red pepper coulis.
- Arrange asparagus beside chicken and sprinkle entire plate with gremolata.
Note: Gremolata is traditionally served over ossu bucco but is a lovely fresh-tasting garnish for any grilled meat.

Per serving: 282 calories, 25 g protein, 33 g carbohydrate, 6 g total fat, 1.3 g fiber, 319 mg sodium
EXCHANGES: 2 vegetable, 2 starch/bread, 2 meat, 1 fat

Salmon au Poivre with Red Wine and Leek Sauce
New Potatoes
Sage and Orange-Steamed Broccoli

4 servings

Ingredients
Sauce
4 Tbsp. ruby port

1 cup finely chopped leeks

4 Tbsp. cabernet (or any dry red wine)

3 Tbsp. rice wine vinegar

1 clove garlic, finely chopped

$1/2$ bay leaf

Fish
4 4-oz. portions of skinless, boneless Atlantic salmon filets

2 tsp. coarsely ground black pepper

Potatoes
2 cups boiled new potatoes

3 fresh sage leaves, julienned

Broccoli
2 cups water

4 cups broccoli

2 Tbsp. chopped orange zest

Assembly
- In a small saucepan, slowly simmer port, leeks, red wine, vinegar, garlic, and bay leaf for 10 minutes, allowing sauce to reduce by one-third.
- Remove bay leaf and set aside.
- Rub pepper into the side of the salmon that formerly had the skin.
- In a hot, nonstick pan sprayed for $1/2$ second with cooking spray, place the salmon, pepper-side-down. Sear for

1 minute and turn. Reduce heat and continue cooking until pink has almost disappeared from the center.
- Boil potatoes and drain; sprinkle with julienned sage.
- Bring water for broccoli to a boil. Add broccoli and orange zest. Cook until tender-crisp. Drain.

Presentation
- Place one salmon filet on each plate.
- Divide leek sauce among all four servings.
- Arrange broccoli and new potatoes alongside.

Per serving: 358 calories, 31 g protein, 43 g carbohydrate, 8 g total fat, 7 g fiber, 102 mg sodium

EXCHANGES: 3 vegetable, 2 starch/bread, 3 meat, $1^{1/2}$ fat

Lettuce-Wrapped Salmon with Fresh Dill and Raspberry Vinaigrette

4 servings

Ingredients
Lettuce

4 quarts water

8 large Romaine lettuce leaves
(unblemished, with no tears)

Fish

4 5-oz. skinless, boneless salmon filets

1/8 tsp. salt

1/8 tsp. black pepper

2 1/2 Tbsp. chopped fresh dill

3 cups water

1 bay leaf

4 black peppercorns

1 Tbsp. olive oil

1 carrot, julienned

1 sweet red pepper, julienned

1 zucchini, julienned

3 stalks celery,* julienned

1 medium onion,* julienned

Other

1/2 cup fat-free raspberry vinaigrette
(store-bought)

Fresh raspberries, for garnish

*Note: Reserve onion peel and celery
trimmings for poaching liquid.

Assembly

- Bring 4 quarts of water to a boil. Gently
place whole Romaine leaves in water.
Allow to cook for 2 minutes. Remove,
carefully placing in large bowl of ice
water. Drain when thoroughly cool.

- Using the flat side of a cleaver or French
knife, gently pound the center rib of the
Romaine leaves 4 to 5 times, until they
become pliable.
- Season salmon filets with salt and pepper.
Sprinkle with fresh dill. Place one
Romaine leaf over each filet, wrapping
the outer edges underneath the filet.
- In a large shallow roasting or saute pan
large enough to accommodate the filets,
bring 3 cups of water to a simmer.
- Add onion *peel* and celery *trimmings*,
bay leaf, and black peppercorns.
- Carefully lower wrapped salmon filets
into the poaching liquid. Cover and
simmer gently for 10 to 12 minutes.
- While salmon is simmering, heat 1
Tbsp. olive oil in large saute pan. Add
julienned carrot, red pepper, zucchini,
celery, and onion. Cook quickly until
tender-crisp.

Presentation
- Scatter the vegetables on four plates.
- Place one salmon filet on each plate and
top each with 2 Tbsp. raspberry vinaigrette.
- Garnish with fresh raspberries.

Per serving: 182 calories, 22 g protein,
12 g carbohydrate, 5 g total fat, 3 g
fiber, 907 mg sodium
EXCHANGES: 2 vegetable, 3 meat, 1 fat

Chef's tips

"Spice up" your own favorite recipes with herbs and herb mixes

Unless dried herbs are specifically called for in a long-cooking sauce or dry seasoning rub, I can't overemphasize the flavor and texture benefits of fresh herbs.

Chop herbs immediately before use to make sure the essential oils don't go to waste. Chopped fresh herbs should be added after cooking or sprinkled on the dish about to be served.

Toss fresh basil and cilantro leaves with your salad greens for a flavor boost.

If you have a sunny window, please try growing your own herbs inside! (Indoor plants do require a sunny location.) In the summer, I keep a planter right outside my kitchen door so it is convenient to snip a few chives or grab a handful of dill.

Some essentials:

Chives	Sage
Basil	Tarragon
Dill	Italian parsley
Thyme	Rosemary
Cilantro	

Create an herb crust by chopping 1/2 cup each spinach, fresh basil, chives, and dill in food processor. Add 1/2 cup toasted bread crumbs; process until fine. Add 2 Tbsp. margarine and blend. Sprinkle over your favorite fish filet and bake. Garnish with orange zest.

Steep 2 Tbsp. chopped fresh tarragon in 1/4 cup dry white wine or vinegar and 1 Tbsp. chopped leeks. Add 1 clove garlic and use as a basting sauce for chicken or fish.

Use wood chips when grilling, or throw on woody stems from tarragon, thyme, or rosemary.

Use 4 Tbsp. balsamic vinegar mixed with 2 Tbsp. of your favorite chopped herbs for a low-cal dressing.

Above all, experiment. You know what *you* like and don't like. Try blending your favorites to make your own "signature" seasonings.

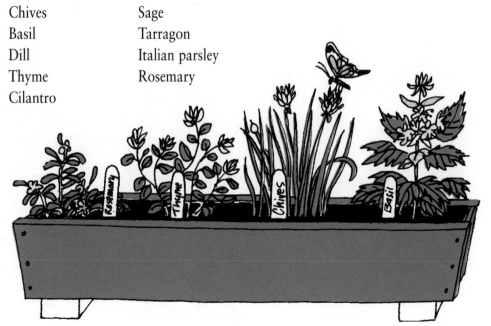

CALCULATIONS AND EQUIVALENTS

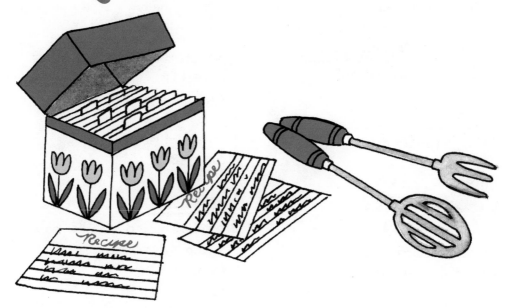

Calculate your own recipes

To calculate the food exchanges in a recipe:

1. List all ingredients and their amounts.

2. For each ingredient, identify the food group and look up the number of exchanges here (or in the exchange lists elsewhere in this book). Sugar in a recipe can be figured as a fruit exchange.

3. Total the number of exchanges in each food group.

4. Divide the total exchanges for each food group by the number of servings the recipe yields. Anything less than one-half of a choice is not counted.

Chocolate

Bitter (baking) 1 oz. = 1 fruit, 3 fat
Chips 1 cup = 4 starch/bread, 7 fat
Cocoa 2 Tbsp. = 1 fat, $1/2$ fruit
Syrup 1 Tbsp. = 1 fruit

Coconut, shredded

$1/4$ cup = 1 fruit, 1 fat
$1/2$ cup = 2 fruit, 2 fat
1 cup = 4 fruit, 4 fat

Cornmeal, dry, uncooked

$1/4$ cup = $1 1/2$ starch/bread

Cornstarch

2 Tbsp. = 1 starch/bread

Flour

$2 1/2$ Tbsp. = 1 starch/bread
$1/4$ cup = $1 1/2$ starch/bread
$1/2$ cup = 3 starch/bread
1 cup = 6 starch/bread

Gelatin, plain, unflavored

1 Tbsp. = $1/2$ meat

Oatmeal, dry, uncooked

1 cup = 4 starch/bread

Marshmallows

1 cup = 1 starch/bread

Pie crust

Crumb $1/6$ 9" pie = 1 starch/bread, 1 fat
Pastry $1/6$ 9" pie = 1 starch/bread, 2 fat

Pasta, dry, uncooked

Macaroni 1 cup = 6 starch/bread
Noodles 1 cup = 4 starch/bread
Spaghetti 1 cup = 8 starch/bread

Rice

Dry, uncooked $1/4$ cup = 2 starch/bread
Instant, dry $1/4$ cup = $1 1/2$ starch/bread
Wild, uncooked $1/4$ cup = $1 1/2$ starch/bread

Shortening

Vegetable shortening, lard, oil, etc.
1 tsp. = 1 fat
1 Tbsp. = 3 fat
$1/4$ cup = 12 fat
$1/2$ cup = 24 fat
1 cup = 48 fat

Sugar

Brown, granulated, molasses, corn syrup
  1 Tbsp. = $1 1/2$ fruit
  $1/4$ cup = 5 fruit
  $1/2$ cup = 10 fruit
  1 cup = 20 fruit
Powdered
  1 Tbsp. = 1 fruit
  $1/4$ cup = 4 fruit
  $1/2$ cup = 8 fruit
  1 cup = 16 fruit

Chopped walnuts

1 Tbsp. = 1 fat
$1/4$ cup = 4 fat
$1/2$ cup = 7 fat, 1 meat
1 cup = 11 fat, 2 meat, $1 1/2$ starch/bread

EQUIVALENTS:
METRIC AND ENGLISH WEIGHTS AND MEASUREMENTS

VOLUME

Measure	English	Metric
1 gallon	4 quarts	3.8 liters
1 quart	2 pints 4 cups 32 fl. ounces	0.95 liter
1.06 quarts	33.8 fl. ounces	1 liter
1 cup	1/2 pint 8 fl. ounces 16 Tbsp.	0.24 liter or 240 milliliters**
1 Tablespoon*	3 teaspoons 1/2 fl. ounce	15 milliliters**
1 teaspoon*	1/8 fl. ounce	5 milliliters**

WEIGHT

Measure	English	Metric
1 pound	16 ounces	0.454 kilogram or 454 grams
2.2 pounds	35.2 ounces	1 kilogram or 1,000 grams
1 ounce	1/16 pound	28.35 grams

* Level measures only
** Milliliters (ml) and cubic centimeters (cc) are often interchanged freely, although this is not strictly correct.

Index

Note: The quizzes and the contents of the 28-Day Guide are not included in this index.